Cardiovascular Disease and Hemodialysis

Cardiovascular Disease and Hemodialysis

Guest Editors

Keren Cohen-Hagai
Moshe Shashar
Sydney Benchetrit

MDPI
Basel • Beijing • Wuhan • Barcelona • Belgrade • Novi Sad • Cluj • Manchester

Guest Editors
Keren Cohen-Hagai
Department of Nephrology and Hypertension
Meir Medical Center
Kfar Saba
Israel

Moshe Shashar
Department of Nephrology and Hypertension
Laniado Hospital
Netanya
Israel

Sydney Benchetrit
Department of Nephrology and Hypertension
Meir Medical Center
Kfar Saba
Israel

Editorial Office
MDPI AG
Grosspeteranlage 5
4052 Basel, Switzerland

This is a reprint of the Special Issue, published open access by the journal *Medicina* (ISSN 1648-9144), freely accessible at: https://www.mdpi.com/journal/medicina/special_issues/780MDJYX1H.

For citation purposes, cite each article independently as indicated on the article page online and as indicated below:

Lastname, A.A.; Lastname, B.B. Article Title. *Journal Name* **Year**, *Volume Number*, Page Range.

ISBN 978-3-7258-5717-3 (Hbk)
ISBN 978-3-7258-5718-0 (PDF)
https://doi.org/10.3390/books978-3-7258-5718-0

Contents

medicina

MDPI

Editorial

Cardiovascular Disease and Hemodialysis

Keren Cohen-Hagai [1,2]

[1] Department of Nephrology and Hypertension, Meir Medical Center, Kfar Saba 4428164, Israel; keren.cohen@clalit.org.il
[2] Gray Faculty of Medical and Health Sciences, Tel Aviv University, Tel Aviv 69978, Israel

Cardiovascular disease (CVD) remains the leading cause of morbidity and mortality in patients undergoing maintenance hemodialysis (HD). The interplay between uremic toxins, vascular calcification, chronic inflammation, malnutrition, and traditional cardiovascular risk factors contributes to a disproportionately high burden of cardiovascular morbidity and mortality in HD population [1–5]. Beyond the clinical implications, this burden carries significant economic consequences for healthcare systems [6]. The persistently elevated and in many settings unacceptable mortality rates in this population reflect not only the complexity of cardiovascular disease pathogenesis in uremia, but also the inadequacy of current preventive and therapeutic strategies [1–5]. These unique pathogenic mechanisms demand focused research efforts and tailored interventions to improve outcomes in this vulnerable group.

This Special Issue of *Medicina*, "Cardiovascular Disease and Hemodialysis", brings together original clinical research that deepens our understanding of the multifaceted cardiovascular burden in this population. The selected studies provide important insights into risk stratification, predictive biomarkers, treatment outcomes, and the pathophysiology of CVD in HD patients.

Nakić et al. evaluated the role of conventional cardiovascular risk factors in dialysis patients with coronary artery disease. Despite the altered metabolic milieu in end-stage kidney disease (ESKD), traditional risk factors such as hypertension, diabetes, and dyslipidemia remained significant contributors to coronary artery disease. This reinforces the relevance of guideline-directed cardiovascular risk factor management in HD patients [7].

LDL cholesterol represents a conventional cardiovascular risk factor that is also addressed in this issue. A retrospective cohort study evaluated the prognostic significance of LDL-C in HD patients hospitalized with acute coronary syndrome (ACS) [8]. Despite similar LDL-C levels and statin use across groups, 30-day and 1-year mortality were significantly higher in HD patients compared to controls. Survival correlated not with LDL-C levels, but with markers of nutrition and inflammation. These findings suggest that in HD patients, inflammation and malnutrition outweigh LDL-C as determinants of post-ACS prognosis [8].

In line with evidence that malnutrition and inflammation outweigh traditional risk factors, Dragoș et al. demonstrated that inflammatory pathways—not solely passive mineral deposition—drive vascular calcification in uremia. This underscores the importance of anti-inflammatory strategies as potential targets in cardiovascular risk mitigation [9]. In ESKD patients, intravascular calcification is both a contributor to and a consequence of CVD. A retrospective study in HD patients found that over 90% had intracranial arterial calcifications (ICACs), markedly higher than among controls [10]. ICAC severity correlated with hypoalbuminemia, hyperphosphatemia, and elevated CRP. In addition, higher ICAC

https://doi.org/10.3390/medicina61101796

scores independently predicted 1-year mortality, highlighting the potential of this measure as a prognostic imaging biomarker in this population.

Wu et al. demonstrated that serum endocan levels, a marker of endothelial activation and inflammation, were significantly associated with increased aortic stiffness in HD patients. The findings provide evidence linking endocan to vascular remodeling and support its utility as a surrogate marker of cardiovascular dysfunction in this group [11]. Šafer et al. explored the prognostic role of endocan in non-diabetic HD patients. Elevated serum endocan predicted adverse cardiovascular events and mortality, further supporting its emerging role as a biomarker of endothelial dysfunction and systemic risk in HD populations [12].

Endothelial dysfunction drives both cardiovascular disease and vascular access complications, both of which significantly affect the prognosis of HD patients. Venegas-Ramírez et al. analyzed long-term survival outcomes in relation to vascular access type. As expected, arteriovenous fistulas (AVFs) were associated with better outcomes compared to catheters. Despite this, AVF utilization remains suboptimal, indicating the need for early referral, vascular mapping, and multidisciplinary planning [13].

The prospective, observational study by Domjanović Matetić et al. examined echocardiographic parameters in ESKD patients undergoing transition from HD to hemodiafiltration (HDF). They found that echocardiographic indices could serve as early markers of cardiovascular adaptation and might inform the timing and benefit of switching to HDF [14].

Dimitrijevic et al. conducted a 24-month cohort study examining bleeding and thrombotic complications in HD patients with atrial fibrillation. Results revealed high rates of both hemorrhagic and thromboembolic events, reflecting the complex and competing risks in this population. These findings call for individualized, risk-adapted antithrombotic strategies for dialysis patients with atrial fibrillation [15].

The studies featured in this Special Issue focusing on cardiovascular disease and hemodialysis collectively emphasize that cardiovascular risk in HD patients is multifactorial, involving not only traditional risk factors but also inflammation, malnutrition, vascular access characteristics, and endothelial dysfunction. Novel biomarkers such as endocan, along with imaging features like ICAC, may aid in refining cardiovascular risk assessment and support evaluating the role of advanced technological options in HD, such as HDF, in controlling and mitigating these processes. Ongoing research is essential to better tailor prevention and treatment strategies to improve survival and quality of life in this vulnerable population.

Funding: This research received no external funding.

Conflicts of Interest: The authors declare no conflict of interest.

References

1. Jankowski, J.; Floege, J.; Fliser, D.; Böhm, M.; Marx, N. Cardiovascular Disease in Chronic Kidney Disease: Pathophysiological Insights and Therapeutic Options. *Circulation* **2021**, *143*, 1157–1172. [CrossRef] [PubMed]
2. Schuett, K.; Marx, N.; Lehrke, M. The Cardio-Kidney Patient: Epidemiology, Clinical Characteristics and Therapy. *Circ. Res.* **2023**, *132*, 902–914. [CrossRef] [PubMed]
3. Schamroth Pravda, M.; Cohen Hagai, K.; Topaz, G.; Schamroth Pravda, N.; Makhoul, N.; Shuvy, M.; Benchetrit, S.; Assali, A.; Pereg, D. Assessment of the CHA2DS2-VASc Score in Predicting Mortality and Adverse Cardiovascular Outcomes of Patients on Hemodialysis. *Am. J. Nephrol.* **2020**, *51*, 635–640. [CrossRef] [PubMed]
4. Einbinder, Y.; Shnaider, A.; Ghanayem, K.; Basok, A.; Rogachev, B.; Lior, Y.; Haviv, Y.S.; Cohen-Hagai, K.; Nacasch, N.; Rozenberg, I.; et al. Elevated Circulating Cell-Free DNA in Hemodialysis-Treated Patients Is Associated with Increased Mortality. *Am. J. Nephrol.* **2020**, *51*, 852–860. [CrossRef] [PubMed]

5. Erez, D.; Fanadka, F.; Benchetrit, S.; Cohen-Hagai, K. The Combined Prognostic Significance of Alkaline Phosphatase and Intracranial Arterial Calcifications in Hemodialysis Patients. *Am. J. Nephrol.* **2021**, *52*, 763–770. [CrossRef] [PubMed]
6. Doan, Q.V.; Gleeson, M.; Kim, J.; Borker, R.; Griffiths, R.; Dubois, R.W. Economic burden of cardiovascular events and fractures among patients with end-stage renal disease. *Curr. Med. Res. Opin.* **2007**, *23*, 1561–1569. [CrossRef] [PubMed]
7. Nakić, D.; Grbić Pavlović, P.; Vojković, M.; Stipćević, M.; Patrk, J.; Bištirlić, M.; Bakotić, Z.; Vučak Lončar, J.; Gusar, I. Coronary Artery Disease in Patients on Dialysis: Impact of Traditional Risk Factors. *Medicina* **2024**, *60*, 1251–1266. [CrossRef] [PubMed]
8. Cohen-Hagai, K.; Benchetrit, S.; Wand, O.; Grupper, A.; Shashar, M.; Solo, O.; Pereg, D.; Zitman-Gal, T.; Haskiah, F.; Erez, D. The Clinical Significance of LDL-Cholesterol on the Outcomes of Hemodialysis Patients with Acute Coronary Syndrome. *Medicina* **2023**, *59*, 1312–1325. [CrossRef] [PubMed]
9. Dragoș, D.; Timofte, D.; Georgescu, M.-T.; Manea, M.-M.; Vacaroiu, I.A.; Ionescu, D.; Balcangiu-Stroescu, A.-E. Cardiovascular Calcifications Are Correlated with Inflammation in Hemodialysis Patients. *Medicina* **2023**, *59*, 1801–1810. [CrossRef] [PubMed]
10. Fanadka, F.; Rozenberg, I.; Nacasch, N.; Einbinder, Y.; Benchetrit, S.; Wand, O.; Hod, T.; Cohen-Hagai, K. Intra-Cranial Arterial Calcifications in Hemodialysis Patients. *Medicina* **2023**, *59*, 1706–1716. [CrossRef] [PubMed]
11. Wu, T.-J.; Wang, C.-H.; Lai, Y.-H.; Kuo, C.-H.; Lin, Y.-L.; Hsu, B.-G. Serum Endocan Is a Risk Factor for Aortic Stiffness in Patients Undergoing Maintenance Hemodialysis. *Medicina* **2024**, *60*, 984–997. [CrossRef] [PubMed]
12. Šafer, M.; Feldi, I.; Šahinović, I.; Tolj, I.; Pirić, M.; Šojat, D.; Oštarijaš, E.; Mihaljević, D. Serum Endocan as a Predictor of Survival and Cardiovascular Events in Patients Without Diabetic Kidney Disease on Chronic Haemodialysis: A Prospective, Observational Study. *Medicina* **2025**, *61*, 991–1005. [CrossRef] [PubMed]
13. Venegas-Ramírez, J.; Hernández-Fuentes, G.A.; Palomares, C.S.; Diaz-Martinez, J.; Navarro-Cuellar, J.I.; Calvo-Soto, P.; Duran, C.; Tapia-Vargas, R.; Espíritu-Mojarro, A.C.; Figueroa-Gutiérrez, A.; et al. Vascular Access Type and Survival Outcomes in Hemodialysis Patients: A Seven-Year Cohort Study. *Medicina* **2025**, *61*, 584–598. [CrossRef] [PubMed]
14. Domjanović Matetić, J.; Baković Kramarić, D.; Domjanović Škopinić, T.; Jeličić, I.; Borić Škaro, D.; Božić, J.; Matetić, A. Echocardiographic Indices in Patients with End-Stage Renal Disease and Their Association with Hemodialysis-to-Hemodiafiltration Transfer: A Prospective Observational Study. *Medicina* **2024**, *60*, 1537–1552. [CrossRef] [PubMed]
15. Dimitrijevic, Z.M.; Mitic, B.P.; Tasic, D.D.; Vrecic, T.; Paunovic, K.; Salinger, S. Bleeding and Thrombotic Events in Hemodialysis Patients with Atrial Fibrillation on Anticoagulation and Antiplatelet Therapy: A 24-Month Cohort Study. *Medicina* **2024**, *60*, 1760–1774. [CrossRef] [PubMed]

medicina MDPI

Article

The Clinical Significance of LDL-Cholesterol on the Outcomes of Hemodialysis Patients with Acute Coronary Syndrome

Keren Cohen-Hagai [1,2,*], Sydney Benchetrit [1,2], Ori Wand [3,4], Ayelet Grupper [2,5], Moshe Shashar [6], Olga Solo [7], David Pereg [8], Tali Zitman-Gal [1,2], Feras Haskiah [2,9] and Daniel Erez [2,9]

1 Department of Nephrology and Hypertension, Meir Medical Center, Kfar Saba 44281, Israel
2 Faculty of Medicine, Tel Aviv University, Tel Aviv 69978, Israel; daniel.erez@clalit.org.il (D.E.)
3 Division of Pulmonary Medicine, Barzilai University Medical Center, Ashkelon 7830604, Israel
4 Faculty of Health Sciences, Ben-Gurion University of the Negev, Beer-Sheva 84105, Israel
5 Department of Nephrology and Hypertension, Tel Aviv Sourasky Medical Center, Tel Aviv 6423906, Israel
6 Department of Nephrology and Hypertension, Laniado Hospital, Netanya 4244916, Israel
7 Department of Anesthesiology, Pain and Intensive Care, Meir Medical Center, Kfar Saba 4428164, Israel
8 Department of Cardiology, Meir Medical Center, Kfar Saba 4428164, Israel
9 Department of Internal Medicine D, Meir Medical Center, Kfar Saba 4428164, Israel
* Correspondence: keren.cohen@clalit.org.il

Abstract: *Background and objectives*: Dyslipidemia is one of the most important modifiable risk factors in the pathogenesis of cardiovascular disease in the general population, but its importance in the hemodialysis (HD) population is uncertain. *Materials and Methods*: This retrospective cohort study includes HD patients hospitalized due to acute coronary syndrome (ACS) in the period 2015–2020 with lipid profile data during ACS. A control group with preserved kidney function was matched. Risk factors for 30-day and 1-year mortality were assessed. *Results*: Among 349 patients included in the analysis, 246 were HD-dependent ("HD group"). HD group patients had higher prevalence of diabetes, hypertension, and heart disease than the control group. At ACS hospitalization, lipid profile and chronic statin treatment were comparable between groups. Odds ratios for 30-day mortality in HD vs. control group was 5.2 (95% CI 1.8–15; $p = 0.002$) and for 1-year, 3.4 (95% CI 1.9–6.1; $p < 0.001$). LDL and LDL < 70 did not change 30-day and 1-year mortality rates in the HD group ($p = 0.995$, 0.823, respectively). However, survival after ACS in HD patients correlated positively with nutritional parameters such as serum albumin ($r = 0.368$, $p < 0.001$) and total cholesterol ($r = 0.185$, $p < 0.001$), and inversely with the inflammatory markers C-reactive protein (CRP; $r = -0.348$, $p < 0.001$) and neutrophils-to-lymphocytes ratio (NLR; $r = -0.181$, $p = 0.019$). Multivariate analysis demonstrated that heart failure was the only significant predictor of 1-year mortality (OR 2.8, $p = 0.002$). LDL < 70 mg/dL at ACS hospitalization did not predict 1-year mortality in the HD group. *Conclusions*: Despite comparable lipid profiles and statin treatment before and after ACS hospitalization, mortality rates were significantly higher among HD group. While malnutrition–inflammation markers were associated with survival of dialysis patients after ACS, LDL cholesterol was not. Thus, our study results emphasize that better nutritional status and less inflammation are associated with improved survival among HD patients.

Keywords: cardiovascular disease; dyslipidemia; LDL cholesterol; hemodialysis; chronic kidney disease

1. Introduction

Chronic kidney disease (CKD) is associated with a marked increase in incidence of mortality from cardiovascular disease (CVD) [1,2]. The annual mortality rate from CVD among patients with end-stage-kidney disease (ESKD) is high and estimated to be over 50% of the overall mortality rate [3–5].

A high level of low-density lipoprotein cholesterol (LDL-C) is a major risk factor for cardiovascular disease among the general population [6], and abnormalities in serum lipid levels associated with renal disease rank high among the factors responsible for accelerated atherosclerosis [7]. Approximately 20–40% of hemodialysis (HD) patients have elevated triglycerides and reduced high-density lipoprotein (HDL) cholesterol levels [8,9]. In addition, increased oxidized LDL-C and increased lipoprotein levels have been reported in up to 75% of HD patients [10]. A meta-analysis of randomized trials undertaken mainly in patients without CKD showed that statin therapy reduces the risk of major coronary events by about one-fifth for each 1 mmol/L reduction in LDL-C [11,12]. However, previous observational data on the effect of LDL-C levels in patients with ESKD yielded conflicting results [13–15]. It has been suggested that as estimated glomerular filtration rate (eGFR) falls below 30 mL/min, a cardiovascular pathophysiology other than accelerated atherosclerosis emerges; and additional variables contribute to the increased rate of cardiovascular events, including oxidative stress, endothelial dysfunction, vascular calcifications and stiffness, sympathetic overactivity [16–18], and malnutrition–inflammation atherosclerosis [19]. The role of inflammation as a risk factor for malnutrition in HD has been recognized in previous trials, and C-reactive protein (CRP) levels have been correlated with the inhibition of albumin synthesis in this particular population [20]. Several observational trials have noted that lower total cholesterol levels are associated with greater mortality in HD patients ("reverse epidemiology") [13,21]. It has been suggested that this paradox results from reverse causation in which advanced cardiovascular disease leads to inflammation, wasting, and lower cholesterol levels, or a confounding effect that results in lower cholesterol levels and increased mortality [22]. In addition, the neutrophils-to-lymphocytes ratio (NLR), a simple biomarker of inflammation, has been shown to predict cardiovascular and all-cause mortality in HD patients [23].

Previous randomized controlled trials which assessed the impact of cholesterol-lowering treatment on cardiovascular outcomes in HD patients have also resulted in conflicting findings [24–26]. While the 4D study [24] and the AURORA study [26] did not detect significant benefits, the SHARP study [25] demonstrated a reduction in major cardiovascular endpoints (MACE) with cholesterol-lowering therapy in a group composed of dialysis and non-dialysis patients. However, the authors mentioned that the study did not have sufficient power to assess the effects on MACE separately in dialysis patients.

Of note, the trials mentioned above did not specifically assess outcomes related to baseline cholesterol levels during acute coronary syndrome (ACS). It has been shown that high-dose statin treatment in ACS patients positively influences the balance between atherogenic and anti-atherogenic lipoproteins in the general population, leading to structural changes in the composition and stability of the atherosclerotic plaque, and producing anti-inflammatory effects and thus improving clinical outcomes [27].

Data regarding baseline cholesterol levels in HD patients during ACS and their relation to adverse cardiovascular outcomes are scarce. The objective of this study was to assess LDL-C levels in a group of HD patients presenting with ACS, and its association with all-cause mortality, compared to patients with normal renal function.

2. Materials and Methods

2.1. Study Design

This retrospective observational study, conducted at Meir Medical Center, evaluated the clinical outcomes of patients hospitalized with a diagnosis of ACS during 2015–2020, with follow-up until 1 January 2021.

Results are reported according to the STROBE statement guidelines.

ACS included all patients with a discharge diagnosis of unstable angina, ST-segment elevation myocardial infarction, or non-ST-segment elevation myocardial infarction.

2.2. Study Population

Our analysis consisted of chronic HD patients treated in the Dialysis Unit at Meir Medical Center from 2015 to 2020, who were hospitalized with a diagnosis of ACS. Chronic HD was defined as at least 3 months of dialysis treatment.

Admission and discharge diagnoses were recorded by the attending physicians based on clinical, electrocardiographic, and biochemical criteria. Mortality data at 30 days and at 1 year post-hospitalization were determined from electronic medical records (EMR) and by the Israeli National Mortality Registry.

The control group was matched to the dialysis group based on age, sex, and hospitalization period. The control group was composed of patients hospitalized with ACS during the same period, who had eGFR > 60 mL/min. EMR were reviewed. Kidney function was assessed using eGFR based on the CKD epidemiology collaboration equation [28].

Patients < 18 years of age or missing EMR data or dialysis vintage < 3 months were excluded, as were subjects treated with PCSK9 inhibitors.

2.3. Variables

Baseline demographic and clinical characteristics of the study patients, including age, sex, medical history of hypertension, diabetes, congestive heart failure, ischemic heart disease, atrial fibrillation, cerebrovascular accident, and peripheral vascular disease were retrieved from the EMR. Laboratory parameters at presentation, including white blood cells (WBC), hemoglobin, platelets, CRP, serum creatinine, urea, albumin, total cholesterol, LDL-C, HDL-C, and triglycerides, were also collected.

NLR was calculated as the ratio of neutrophils-to-lymphocytes from the differential white blood cell count routinely evaluated at the beginning of dialysis sessions.

2.4. Ethical Considerations

The study was approved by the Institutional Ethics Committee in keeping with the principles of the Declaration of Helsinki. In accordance with Ministry of Health regulations, the Institutional Ethics Committee did not require written informed consent because data were collected anonymously from the EMR without active patient participation.

2.5. Statistical Analysis

Data are presented as numbers and percentages for nominal parameters and as means and standard deviations for continuous parameters. Differences between the study groups were analyzed using the chi-square test. Continuous variables were analyzed using the one-way ANOVA test. Spearman correlation was calculated to assess correlation between continuous variables. A multivariate logistic regression model including all significant variables in the univariate analysis was applied to estimate odds ratios. Multivariate models for predicting mortality were conducted using logistic regression analysis comparing 30-day and 1-year mortality rates by kidney function group (the control group with eGFR >60 mL/min served as the reference group). The HD group was compared to the control group. Kaplan–Meier survival curve analysis was performed in order to detect differences in survival of HD patients following ACS when comparing by LDL-C. $p < 0.05$ was considered statistically significant.

Data were analyzed with SPSS Version 27 (IBM Corporation, Armonk, NY, USA).

3. Results

This retrospective analysis included 349 patients, among which 246 were defined as chronic dialysis patients prior to hospitalization for ACS (HD group).

Baseline demographic and clinical characteristics of the patients are summarized in Table 1. HD patients had higher prevalence of diabetes, hypertension, heart failure, ischemic heart disease, peripheral vascular disease, and atrial fibrillation. They also had lower hemoglobin levels compared to the control group.

Table 1. Baseline demographic and clinical characteristics of study groups.

Variable	HD Group (N = 246)	Control Group (N = 103)	*p*-Value
Age, years; mean ± SD	72.4 ± 10.5	71.3 ± 11.8	0.68
Male sex, n (%)	168 (68.3)	66 (64.1)	0.45
Diabetes, n (%)	159 (64.9)	40 (40.8)	<0.01
Ischemic heart disease, n (%)	175 (71.1)	44 (44.9)	<0.01
Heart failure, n (%)	83 (33.7)	12 (12.2)	<0.01
Hypertension, n (%)	231 (93.9)	67 (68.4)	<0.01
Previous stroke, n (%)	53 (21.5)	9 (9.2)	<0.01
Atrial fibrillation, n (%)	43 (17.6)	8 (8.2)	0.03
Peripheral vascular disease, n (%)	57 (23.2)	6 (6.2)	<0.001
Laboratory tests at admission for ACS hospitalization			
WBC (K/microl)	9.8 ± 7.9	10.4 ± 5.6	0.48
Hemoglobin (g/dL)	10.4 ± 1.7	12.7 ± 2.1	<0.01
Platelets (K/microl)	234 ± 110	246 ± 87	0.34
Neutrophil to lymphocyte ratio	9 ± 10.6	7.4 ± 10.9	0.22
C-reactive protein (mg/dL)	7.9 ± 17.5	2.6 ± 4.7	0.01
Serum creatinine (mg/dL)	5.2 ± 11.8	1.1 ± 1	<0.01
Urea (mg/dL)	118.9 ± 60.5	43.7 ± 18.1	<0.01
Albumin(g/dL)	3.4 ± 2.3	3.7 ± 0.5	0.71
Total cholesterol (mg/dL)	153.1 ± 58.1	168 ± 55.2	0.03
HDL-C (mg/dL)	37.9 ± 14.3	40.6 ± 11.1	0.21
Triglycerides (mg/dL)	147.5 ± 80.2	157.2 ± 97.9	0.46
LDL-C (mg/dL)	77.2 ± 41.8	87.4 ± 36.1	0.11

HD, hemodialysis; HDL-C, high density lipoprotein cholesterol; LDL-C, low density lipoprotein cholesterol.

3.1. LDL-C in the HD Group

LDL-C levels were normally distributed. Average and median LDL-C levels at admission were similar for the HD and control groups. (Table 1 and Figure 1).

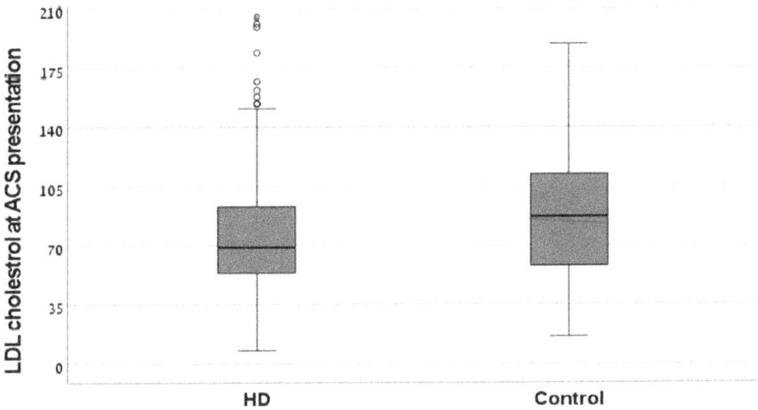

Figure 1. Box plot of LDL-C levels at acute coronary syndrome (ACS) presentation. Box-plot describing median, 25th, and 75th percentile, and minimum and maximum levels of LDL-C (mg/dL) at ACS presentation. The median LDL-C level at ACS presentation was 69 in the HD group and 87 in the control group.

Eighty HD patients had LDL-C < 70 mg/dL (32.5%) versus 16 subjects (15.5%) in the control group ($p < 0.01$, Table 2). Despite a higher prevalence of LDL-C < 70 mg/dl in the HD group, rates of statin treatment before and after ACS hospitalization were comparable between groups (Table 2).

Table 2. LDL-C and statin treatment in study groups.

Variable	HD Group N = 246	Control Group N = 103	*p*-Value
LDL-C (mg/dL), mean ± SD	77.2 ± 41.8	87.4 ± 36.1	0.11
LDL-C < 70 mg/dL, N (%)	80 (32.5)	16 (15.5)	<0.01
Statin treatment before, N (%)	175 (71.1)	61 (59.2)	0.14
Statin treatment after, N (%)	212 (86.2)	84 (81.6)	0.92

LDL-C, low density lipoprotein cholesterol.

3.2. 30-Day Mortality

Among the 349 patients in this cohort, 47 died within 30-days after ACS admission. The 30-day mortality rate was higher in the HD group (43 patients, 17.5%) vs. the control group (four patients, 3.9%, $p < 0.01$). OR for 30-day mortality in the HD group was 5.2 (95% CI 1.8–15) vs. control group (Table 3).

Table 3. Odds ratio for mortality in study groups.

Coefficients	Odds Ratio	95% Confidence Interval Lower	Upper	*p*-Value
30-day mortality				
Control group		Reference		
HD group	5.2	1.8	15	<0.01
1-year mortality				
Control group		Reference		
HD group	3.4	1.9	6.1	<0.01

HD, hemodialysis. Low LDL-C (<70 mg/dL) did not predict the 30-day mortality rate in the HD group ($p = 0.995$); the 30-day mortality was 17.5% for both HD patients with LDL-C < 70 mg/dL (14/80) and for those with LDL-C ≥ 70 mg/dL (29/166).

3.3. One-Year Mortality

In the HD group, 99 patients (40.2%) died within 1 year as compared to 16.5% in the control group ($p < 0.001$). OR for 1-year mortality in the HD group was 3.4 (95% CI 1.9–6.1) vs. the control group (Table 3).

One-year mortality rates were similar for HD patients with LDL-C < 70 mg/dL: 33/80, 41.3%, and those with LDL-C ≥ 70 mg/dL, 66/166, 39.8%, $p = 0.82$. Similarly, low LDL-C (<70 mg/dL) was not associated with survival rates over time in the HD group ($p = 0.503$; Figure 2).

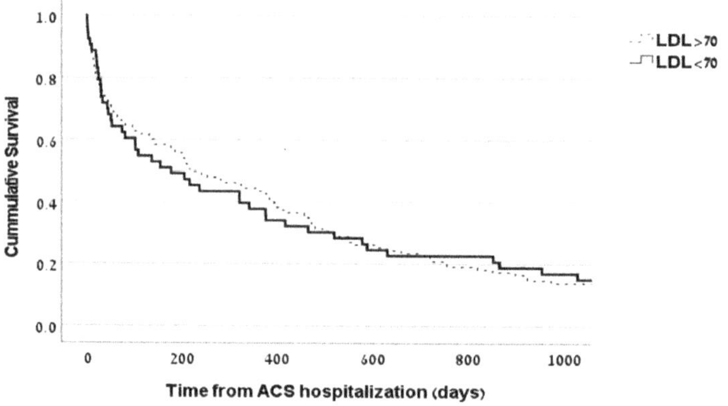

Figure 2. Survival rate in HD group according to LDL-C level. Kaplan–Meier survival curve did not demonstrate differences in survival of HD patients following ACS when comparing by LDL-C ($p = 0.503$). HD, hemodialysis; ACS, acute coronary syndrome; LDL-C, low density lipoprotein cholesterol.

3.4. Predictors of Mortality after ACS in HD Group

As mentioned above, mortality rates were significantly higher among HD vs. control patients both at 30-day and 1-year mortality after ACS, and rates of statin treatment were comparable between HD and control group both before and after ACS hospitalization. There was also no correlation between LDL-C levels and mortality rates (r = 0.1, $p = 0.321$). Among HD patients, 1-year survival after ACS was positively associated with the nutritional parameters of serum albumin (r = 0.368, $p < 0.001$) and total cholesterol (r = 0.185, $p < 0.018$). Survival was inversely correlated with the inflammatory markers CRP (r = −0.348, $p < 0.001$) and NLR; (r = −0.181, $p = 0.019$). Dialysis vintage was not significantly correlated with survival after ACS (r = −0.161, $p = 0.125$).

Multivariate analysis demonstrated that heart failure was the only significant predictor for 1-year mortality (OR 2.8, $p = 0.002$, Table 4). Low LDL-C (<70 mg/dL) at ACS hospitalization did not predict 1-year mortality in the HD group.

Table 4. Multivariate analysis model for 1-year mortality in HD group (n = 246).

Coefficients	Odds Ratio	95% Confidence Interval Lower	95% Confidence Interval Upper	p-Value
Female sex	0.907	0.489	1.681	0.756
Diabetes	0.783	0.436	1.406	0.413
Ischemic heart disease	1.633	0.865	3.083	0.13
Heart failure	2.765	1.468	5.208	0.002
Previous stroke	0.628	0.316	1.247	0.183
Atrial fibrillation	1.437	0.678	3.044	0.344
Peripheral vascular disease	0.748	0.38	1.469	0.399
LDL-C < 70 (mg/dL)	1.175	0.658	2.098	0.587

4. Discussion

This retrospective analysis found increased mortality among HD patients presenting with ACS compared to a control group matched for age and sex, yet with a normal eGFR. This was despite numerically lower median LDL-C levels at presentation and similar rates of statin prescription, both at presentation and at discharge. Moreover, a significant proportion of HD patients had LDL-C < 70 mg/dL; however, this parameter did not affect survival among the HD group at both 30-day and 1-year time points.

The finding of increased mortality among HD patients after ACS hospitalization is not surprising; it is well-established as cardiovascular disease is a leading cause of death in this population. Cardiovascular pathophysiology in CKD patients consists of traditional risk-factors (diabetes, dyslipidemia, hypertension), as well as mediators promoting vascular calcification [29]. For example, reduced kidney function and albuminuria are associated with an increase in cardiovascular risk and are independent of these traditional risk factors. In fact, there is an inverse non-linear relationship between eGFR and cardiovascular events, with HD patients experiencing 10- to 30-fold higher CV mortality risk [2,30].

Qualitative abnormalities in serum lipids associated with renal disease rank high among the factors responsible for accelerated atherosclerosis [6]. Thus, the increased prevalence of CVD in patients with ESKD is not necessarily due to elevated LDL-C. More frequently, chylomicrons remnants and high-density lipoprotein deficiency and dysfunction are involved in the increased atherosclerosis observed in ESKD patients. Dyslipidemia and low grade inflammation are also caused by chronic kidney disease [31]. In patients with impaired kidney function, lipid profiles become atherogenic, partly due to defective HDL-C function and excessive oxidation of LDL-C [32]. Mechanisms responsible for systemic inflammation in CKD are incompletely understood. However, increased production of inflammatory mediators has been attributed to raised oxidative stress and accumulation of post-synthetically modified proteins and toxins that are cleared with normal renal function [33].

While older observational studies showed improved survival in HD patients receiving HMG-CoA reductase inhibitors (statins), recent randomized controlled trials yielded conflicting results [24–26]. The role of PCSK9 inhibitors in this population has not yet been elucidated. Major prospective studies on patients not undergoing percutaneous coronary intervention (PCI) or upon presentation with ACS have examined the impact of decreased LDL-C on cardiovascular outcomes in HD patients. In the AURORA trial [26], in which 2776 HD patients were divided into a placebo group and a treatment group receiving 10 mg/day rosuvastatin, the combined outcome of cardiovascular death, non-fatal MI, or non-fatal cerebrovascular disorder was not significantly reduced in the treatment group. Similarly, the 4D study [24], which consisted of 1255 HD patients with diabetes mellitus, did not demonstrate a significant reduction in major cardiovascular endpoints in patients receiving 20 mg/day of atorvastatin.

The SHARP study [25] included 9720 patients with CKD (33% on HD). After 5 years of follow-up, combination therapy of simvastatin plus ezetimibe reduced the incidence of major cardiovascular outcomes for the whole cohort. The authors postulated that the failure to achieve significance in the AURORA and 4D studies might derive from the much smaller numbers and proportions of modifiable cardiovascular events in those studies. Of note, the subgroup of HD patients in the SHARP study showed no benefit with treatment. It was mentioned that the study did not have sufficient power to assess the effects on MACE separately in dialysis patients.

In contrast to those studies, information regarding factors related to adverse outcomes, including baseline LDL-C levels, in HD patients presenting with ACS is limited, despite the fact that ACS treatment has progressed significantly in the current era with the use of anti-aggregates, anti-diabetics, and lipid-lowering drugs. The Collaborative Atorvastatin Diabetes Study (CARDS) reported decreased cardiovascular death among patients with type 2 diabetes mellitus treated with atorvastatin in the absence of marked renal insufficiency [34]. However, CKD is still associated with short- and long-term adverse outcomes in patients with cardiovascular disease. While shared risk factors and a sustained inflammatory state may explain this increased risk, guidelines recommending therapies, including statin treatment, are still underutilized [35].

Nagata et al. [36] evaluated factors associated with MACE in HD patients undergoing PCI without ACS compared to a control group of non-HD patients. It was shown that the risk of MACE in HD decreased as LDL-C increased, in contrast to the control group. However, as mentioned, the trial consisted of patients undergoing elective PCI.

Shechter et al. [37] assessed the impact of statin therapy on patients presenting with ACS. They found an inverse correlation between eGFR and statin prescription at discharge. In addition, CKD patients not prescribed statins experienced higher mortality rates. Of note, only 6% of the study population had an eGFR < 30 mL/min, and it was not mentioned whether HD patients were included in the study. In addition, LDL-C levels at admission and the rate of statin usage prior to hospitalization were not assessed.

In our study, more than 50% of the participants were HD patients, potentially enabling better assessment of this specific population. Our analysis showed similar rates of statin administration, both at admission and discharge, between HD patients and the control group. Moreover, median LDL-C levels were lower in the HD group. Low levels of serum total cholesterol in subjects on HD may indicate the presence of malnutrition and are often associated with hypoalbuminemia. Hypocholesterolemia is common in chronic dialysis patients, yet its mechanisms are not well delineated. Cytokinemia related to impaired removal of substances or to exposure to occult chronic inflammation may be involved in the pathogenesis [38]. Declining serum cholesterol levels in HD patients may be an indicator of either declining health or metabolic, dietary, and other clinical abnormalities similar to those associated with old age [39]. Iseki et al. [13] demonstrated a significant correlation between serum cholesterol and albumin levels. In fact, high serum cholesterol levels were an independent predictor of death in a subgroup of patients with relatively high albumin levels. However, a significant proportion of hypocholesterolemic patients in their study had elevated CRP levels. It has been suggested that the paradoxical association between lipid levels and outcomes in HD patients results from either reverse causation, in which advanced cardiovascular disease leads to inflammation, wasting, and lower cholesterol levels, or a confounding effect resulting in lower cholesterol levels and increased mortality [40]. Whereas LDL-C in our cohort did not seem to play a crucial role in the outcomes of HD patients hospitalized due to ACS, our results emphasize the importance of inflammation and malnutrition in their prognosis. Previous trials [13,22] have demonstrated that in the absence of inflammation, the relationship between total cholesterol level (not LDL-C) and mortality in HD patients is the same as in the general population. In a post hoc analysis of the 4D study, Krane et al. [40] examined the combined significance of LDL-C and CRP (as a marker of inflammation) in predicting cardiovascular outcomes among HD patients. They concluded that CRP level is more important than LDL-C in predicting the risk of death and cardiovascular events in those patients. In addition, low albumin, a marker of inflammation and malnutrition, has been shown to increase susceptibility to infection and death in HD patients [41].

Recently, NLR has emerged as a surrogate marker for systemic inflammation in CKD and HD patients [23,42,43]. It is a cost-effective and simple parameter, allowing for the easily assessment of the inflammatory status of a subject, especially in settings where CRP is not measured routinely [44]. It has been shown to be a strong and independent predictor of cardiovascular severity and mortality in maintenance HD patients [45]. Erdem et al. [46] also reported the usefulness of NLR in predicting short-term mortality among patients receiving HD in hospital settings. In a study assessing the relationship of NLR with nutritional markers and outcomes in HD patients, Diaz et al. [23] demonstrated that low NLR levels were associated with decreased hospitalization rate. Although their trial did not reach statistical significance for reduced mortality rates related to low NLR levels, no fatal outcomes occurred in the lowest NLR quartile, while all deaths registered during the study period occurred in the higher NLR quartile. These results support those achieved in other studies. Although baseline NLR did not differ between the control group and the HD group in our study, survival following ACS was significantly associated with increased NLR, thus supporting the findings of previous studies.

We believe our study contributes to the literature by specifically examining the impact of LDL-C at admission with ACS in a large group of HD patients compared to a control group hospitalized at the same time and at the same institute. We also showed that the use of statins was not different between the groups at both hospital admission and discharge. This parameter has important clinical implications since according to current guidelines [47,48], statins are commonly prescribed at discharge following ACS. Our results, in concordance with previous studies, emphasize the importance of nutritional and inflammatory parameters, including albumin, total cholesterol, CRP, and NLR, in predicting clinical outcomes of HD patients following diagnosis of ACS. Thus, nephrologists and healthcare providers of dialysis patients should make every effort to improve the nutritional status of these patients. Since our study did not demonstrate a survival difference related to LDL-C levels above or below 70 mg/dL in HD patients, it would have been interesting to evaluate whether inflammatory and nutritional markers, including CRP, NLR, total cholesterol, and serum albumin, differed between these two groups, thus affecting clinical outcomes. Unfortunately, due to its retrospective design, such a causative association could not be determined in our study.

Our study also had several limitations inherent to its retrospective design and use of electronic databases. Information regarding statin treatment was based on admission and discharge letters. We did not perform regular follow-up on the continuation of statin treatment following discharge in the study population, and we did not differentiate between different statin types or dosages. Since attending nephrologists frequently withhold statin treatment in HD patients, this could potentially influence final outcomes. We also did not collect data regarding glycemic control and treatment or the prescription of other cardioprotective agents following ACS, such as beta blockers, renin-angiotensin system inhibitors (RASI), and sodium glucose 2 transporter (SGLT-2) inhibitors, which are associated with improved survival following ACS. Since a substantial portion of these drugs are either under-used or contraindicated in hemodialysis patients, this could affect prognosis in the study group.

Nevertheless, we believe our results are important since they highlight the value of regular surveillance of inflammatory and nutritional parameters in HD patients presenting with ACS.

5. Conclusions

Our study found decreased one-year survival in HD patients presenting with ACS compared to a group of non-dialysis patients with preserved kidney function despite a lower median LDL-C level at diagnosis and similar usage of statin treatment both at diagnosis and discharge. Among the HD group, survival was mainly related to easily measured inflammatory and nutritional parameters. Frequent clinical surveillance is warranted in HD patients at increased risk for mortality following ACS.

Author Contributions: Research area and study design: D.P., S.B., O.W. and K.C.-H.; Data acquisition: D.E., O.S., T.Z.-G., F.H. and K.C.-H.; Data analysis and interpretation: S.B., O.W., D.P., D.E., A.G., M.S. and K.C.-H.; Statistical analysis: S.B. and K.C.-H.; Supervision or mentorship: D.E., S.B. and K.C.-H. Each author contributed important intellectual content during manuscript drafting or revision and agrees to be personally accountable for the individual's own contributions. All authors have read and agreed to the published version of the manuscript.

Funding: This research received no external funding.

Institutional Review Board Statement: The study was conducted in accordance with the Declaration of Helsinki and approved by the Institutional Review Board of Meir Medical Center (MMC-0359-20, was approved in 15 December 2020).

Informed Consent Statement: Patient consent was waived due to the retrospective design of the study.

Data Availability Statement: All data analyzed during this study are included in this article. Further enquiries can be directed to the corresponding author.

Acknowledgments: We thank Faye Schreiber, for editing the manuscript. She is an employee of Meir Medical Center.

Conflicts of Interest: The authors have no financial or other conflict of interest to declare.

References

1. Matsushita, K.; Van der Velde, M.; Astor, B.C.; Woodward, M.; Levey, A.S.; De Jong, P.E.; Coresh, J.; Gansevoort, R.T.; Chronic Kidney Disease Prognosis Consortium. Association of estimated glomerular filtration rate and albuminuria with all-cause and cardiovascular mortality in general population cohorts: A collaborative meta-analysis. *Lancet* **2010**, *375*, 2073–2081.
2. Haim-Pinhas, H.; Yoskovitz, G.; Lishner, M.; Pereg, D.; Kitay-Cohen, Y.; Topaz, G.; Sela, Y.; Wand, O.; Rozenberg, I.; Benchetrit, S.; et al. Effect of aspirin on primary prevention of cardiovascular disease and mortality among patients with chronic kidney disease. *Sci. Rep.* **2022**, *12*, 17788. [CrossRef]
3. US Renal Data System. USRDS 1999 annual data report. *Am. J. Kidney Dis.* **1999**, *34* (Suppl. 1), S87–S94.
4. Schamroth-Pravda, M.; Cohen-Hagai, K.; Topaz, G.; Schamroth-Pravda, N.; Makhoul, N.; Shuvy, M.; Benchetrit, S.; Assali, A.; Pereg, D. Assessment of the CHA2DS2-VASc Score in Predicting Mortality and Adverse Cardiovascular Outcomes of Patients on Hemodialysis. *Am. J. Nephrol.* **2020**, *51*, 635–640. [CrossRef] [PubMed]
5. Cohen-Hagai, K.; Nacasch, N.; Rozenberg, I.; Korzets, Z.; Einbinder, Y.; Zitman-Gal, T.; Benchetrit, S. Clinical outcomes of stroke in hemodialysis patients: A retrospective single-center study. *Int. Urol. Nephrol.* **2019**, *51*, 1435–1441. [CrossRef] [PubMed]
6. Grundy, S.M.; Stone, N.; Bailey, A.L.; Beam, C.; Birtcher, K.K.; Blumenthal, R.S.; Braun, L.T.; De Ferranti, S.; Faiella-Tommasino, J.; Forman, D.E.; et al. Guideline on the management of blood cholesterol: Executive summary: A report of the American college of cardiology/American heart association task force on clinical practice guidelines. *J. Am. Coll. Cardiol.* **2019**, *73*, 3168–3209. [CrossRef] [PubMed]
7. Prichard, S.S. Impact of dyslipidemia in end-stage renal disease. *J. Am. Soc. Nephrol.* **2003**, *14* (Suppl. 4), S315–S320. [CrossRef] [PubMed]
8. Avram, M.M.; Goldwasser, P.; Burrell, D.E.; Antignani, A.; Fein, P.A.; Mittman, N. The uremic dyslipidemia: A cross-sectional and longitudinal study. *Am. J. Kidney Dis.* **1992**, *20*, 324–335. [CrossRef]

9. Elisof, M.; Mikhailidis, D.P.; Siampoulos, K.C. Dyslipidemia in patients with renal disease. *J. Drug Dev. Clin. Pr.* **1996**, *17*, 331–348.
10. Kronenberg, F.; König, P.; Neyer, U.; Auinger, M.; Pribasnig, A.; Lang, U.; Reitinger, J.; Pinter, G.; Utermann, G.; Dieplinger, H. Multicenter study of lipoprotein(a) and apolipoprotein(a) phenotypes in patients with end-stage renal disease treated with hemodialysis or continuous ambulatory peritoneal dialysis. *J. Am. Soc. Nephrol.* **1995**, *6*, 110–120. [CrossRef]
11. Cholesterol Treatment Trialists (CTT) Collaboration. Efficacy and safety of more intensive lowering of LDL cholesterol: A meta-analysis of data from 170,000 participants in 26 randomized trials. *Lancet* **2010**, *376*, 1670–1681. [CrossRef] [PubMed]
12. Cholesterol Treatment Trialists (CTT) Collaboration. Efficacy and safety of cholesterol-lowering treatment: Prospective meta-analysis of data from 90,056 participants in 14 randomized trials of statins. *Lancet* **2005**, *366*, 1267–1278. [CrossRef] [PubMed]
13. Iseki, K.; Yamazato, M.; Tozawa, M.; Takishita, S. Hypocholesterolemia is a significant predictor of death in a cohort of chronic hemodialysis patients. *Kidney Int.* **2002**, *61*, 1887–1893. [CrossRef]
14. Seliger, S.L.; Weiss, N.S.; Gillen, D.L.; Kestenbaum, B.; Ball, A.; Sherrard, D.J.; Stehman-Breen, C.O. HMG-CoA reductase inhibitors are associated with reduced mortality in ESRD patients. *Kidney Int.* **2002**, *61*, 297–304. [CrossRef] [PubMed]
15. Mason, N.A.; Bailie, G.R.; Satayathum, S.; Bragg-Gresham, J.L.; Akiba, T.; Akizawa, T.; Combe, C.; Rayner, H.C.; Saito, A.; Gillespie, B.W.; et al. HMGCoA reductase inhibitor use is associated with mortality reduction in hemodialysis patients. *Am. J. Kidney Dis.* **2005**, *45*, 119–126. [CrossRef]
16. Amann, K.; Breitbach, M.; Ritz, E.; Mall, G. Myocyte/capillary mismatch in the heart of uremic patients. *J. Am. Soc. Nephrol.* **1998**, *9*, 1018–1022. [CrossRef]
17. Einbinder, Y.; Shnaider, A.; Ghanayem, K.; Basok, A.; Rogachev, B.; Lior, Y.; Haviv, Y.S.; Cohen-Hagai, K.; Nacasch, N.; Rozenberg, I.; et al. Elevated Circulating Cell-Free DNA in Hemodialysis-Treated Patients Is Associated with Increased Mortality. *Am. J. Nephrol.* **2020**, *51*, 852–860. [CrossRef]
18. Erez, D.; Fanadka, F.; Benchetrit, S.; Cohen-Hagai, K. The Combined Prognostic Significance of Alkaline Phosphatase and Intracranial Arterial Calcifications in Hemodialysis Patients. *Am. J. Nephrol.* **2021**, *52*, 763–770. [CrossRef]
19. Choi, S.R.; Lee, Y.K.; Cho, A.J.; Park, H.C.; Han, C.H.; Choi, M.J.; Koo, J.R.; Yoon, J.W.; Noh, J.W. Malnutrition, inflammation, progression of vascular calcification and survival: Inter-relationships in hemodialysis patients. *PLoS ONE* **2019**, *14*, e0216415. [CrossRef]
20. Kaysen, G.A.; Chertow, G.M.; Adhikarla, R.; Young, B.; Ronco, C.; Levin, N.W. Inflammation and dietary protein intake exert competing effects on serum albumin and creatinine in hemodialys patients. *Kidney Int.* **2001**, *60*, 333–340. [CrossRef]
21. Chiang, C.-K.; Ho, T.-I.; Hsu, S.-P.; Peng, Y.-S.; Pai, M.-F.; Yang, S.-Y.; Hung, K.-Y.; Tsai, T.-J. Low-density lipoprotein cholesterol: Association with mortality and hospitalization in hemodialysis patients. *Blood Purif.* **2005**, *23*, 134–140. [CrossRef] [PubMed]
22. Liu, Y.; Coresh, J.; Eustace, J.A.; Longenecker, J.C.; Jaar, B.; Fink, N.E.; Tracy, R.P.; Powe, N.R.; Klag, M.J. Association between cholesterol level and mortality in dialysis patients: Role of inflammation and malnutrition. *JAMA* **2004**, *291*, 451–459. [CrossRef] [PubMed]
23. Diaz-Martinez, J.; Campa, A.; Delgado-Enciso, I.; Hain, D.; George, F.; Huffman, F.; Baum, M. The relationship of blood lymphocute-to-neutrophil ratio with nutritional markers and health outcomes in hemodialysis patients. *Int. Urol. Nephrol.* **2019**, *51*, 1239–1247. [CrossRef] [PubMed]
24. Wanner, C.; Krane, V.; März, W.; Olschewski, M.; Mann, J.F.; Ruf, G.; Ritz, E. Atorvastatin in patients with type 2 diabetes mellitus undergoing hemodialysis. *N. Engl. J. Med.* **2005**, *353*, 238–248. [CrossRef] [PubMed]
25. Baignet, C.; Landray, M.J.; Reith, C.; Emberson, J.; Wheeler, D.C.; Tomson, C.; Wanner, C.; Krane, V., Cass, A.; Craig, J.; et al. The effects of lowering LDL cholesterol with simvastatin plus ezetimibe in patients with chronic kidney disease (study of heart and renal protection): A randomized placebo-controlled trial. *Lancet* **2011**, *377*, 2181–2192. [CrossRef]
26. Fellström, B.C.; Jardine, A.G.; Schmieder, R.E.; Holdaas, H.; Bannister, K.; Beutler, J.; Chae, D.-W.; Chevaile, A.; Cobbe, S.M.; Grönhagen-Riska, C.; et al. Rosuvastatin and cardiovascular events in patients undergoing hemodialysis. *N. Engl. J. Med.* **2009**, *360*, 1395–1407. [CrossRef]
27. Sposito, A.C.; Chapman, M.J. Statin therapy in acute coronary syndromes, mechanistic insight into clinical benefit. *Arter. Thromb. Vasc. Biol.* **2002**, *22*, 1524–1534. [CrossRef]
28. Levey, A.S.; Stevens, L.A.; Schmid, C.H.; Zhang, Y.L.; Castro, A.F., 3rd; Feldman, H.I.; Kusek, J.W.; Eggers, P.; Van Lente, F.; Greene, T.; et al. CKD-EPI (Chronic Kidney Disease Epidemiology Collaboration). *New Equ. Estim. Glomerular Filtr. Rate. Ann. Intern. Med.* **2009**, *5*, 604–612.
29. Gansevoort, R.T.; Correa-Rotter, R.; Hemmelgarn, B.R.; Jafar, T.H.; Heerspink, H.J.; Mann, J.F.; Matsushita, K.; Wen, C.P. Chronic kidney disease and cardiovascular risk: Epidemiology, mechanisms and prevention. *Lancet* **2013**, *382*, 339–352. [CrossRef]
30. Go, A.S.; Chertow, G.M.; Fan, D.; McCulloch, C.E.; Hsu, C. Chronic kidney disease and the risks of death, cardiovascular events, and hospitalizations. *N. Eng. J. Med.* **2004**, *351*, 1295–1305. [CrossRef]
31. Krane, V.; Wanner, C. Statins, inflammation and kidney disease. *Nat. Rev. Nephrol.* **2011**, *6*, 1573–1579. [CrossRef] [PubMed]
32. Bakris, G.L. Lipid disorders in uremia and dialysis. *Contrib. Nephrol.* **2012**, *178*, 100–105. [PubMed]
33. Schiffrin, E.L.; Lipman, M.L.; Mann, J.F.E. Chronic kidney disease: Effects on the cardiovascular system. *Circulation* **2007**, *116*, 85–97. [CrossRef] [PubMed]

34. Colhoun, H.M.; Betteridge, D.J.; Durrington, P.N.; Hitman, G.A.; Neil HA, W.; Livingstone, S.J.; Thomason, M.J.; Mackness, M.I.; Charlton-Menys, V.; Fuller, J.H.; et al. Primary prevention of cardiovascular disease with atorvastatin in type 2 diabetes in the Collaborative Atorvastatin Diabetes Study (CARDS) multicenter randomized placebo-controlled trial. *Lancet* **2004**, *364*, 685–696. [CrossRef] [PubMed]
35. Tonelli, M.; Bohm, C.; Pandeya, S.; Gill, J.; Levin, A.; Kiberd, B.A. Cardiac risk factors and the use of cardioprotective medications in patients with chronic renal insufficiency. *Am. J. Kidney Dis.* **2001**, *37*, 484–489. [CrossRef]
36. Nagata, I.; Ike, A.; Nishikawa, H.; Zhang, B.; Sugihara, M.; Mori, K.; Iwata, A.; Kawamura, A.; Shirai, K.; Uehara, Y.; et al. Associations beween lipid profile and MACE in hemodialysis patients with percutaneous coronary intervention: From the FU-Registry. *J. Cardiol.* **2015**, *65*, 105–111. [CrossRef]
37. Natanzon, S.S.; Matetzky, S.; Beigel, R.; Iakobishvili, Z.; Goldenberg, I.; Shechter, M. Statin therapy among chronic kidney disease patients presenting with acute coronary syndrome. *Atherosclerosis* **2019**, *286*, 14–19. [CrossRef]
38. Bologa, R.M.; Levine, D.M.; Parker, T.S.; Cheigh, J.S.; Serur, D.; Stenzel, K.H.; Rubin, A.L. Interleukin-6 predicts hypoalbuminemia, hypocholesterolemia and mortality in hemodialysis patients. *Am. J. Kidney Dis.* **1998**, *32*, 107–114. [CrossRef]
39. Pekkanen, J.; Nissinen, A.; Vartiainen, E.; Salonen, J.T.; Punsar, S.; Karvonen, M.J. Changes in serum cholesterol level and mortality: A 30-year followup. The finish cohorts of the sevne countries study. *Am. J. Epidemiol.* **1994**, *139*, 155–165. [CrossRef]
40. Krane, V.; Winkler, K.; Drechsler, C.; Lilienthal, J.; Marz, W.; Wanner, C. Association of LDL cholesterol and inflammation with cardiovascular events and mortality in patients with type 2 diabetes mellitus. *Am. J. Kidney Dis.* **2009**, *54*, 902–911. [CrossRef]
41. Pecoits-Filho, R.; Lindholm, B.; Stenvinkel, P. The malnutrition, inflammation, and atherosclerosis (MIA) syndrome. *Nephrol. Dial. Transpl.* **2002**, *17*, 28–31. [CrossRef] [PubMed]
42. Okyay, G.U.; İnal, S.; Öneç, K.; Er, R.E.; Paşaoğlu, Ö.; Paşaoğlu, H.; Derici, Ü.; Erten, Y. Neutrophil to lymphocyte ratio in evaluation of inflammation in patients with chronic kidney disease. *Ren. Fail.* **2013**, *35*, 29–36. [CrossRef] [PubMed]
43. Turkmen, K.; Guney, I.; Yerlikaya, F.H.; Tonbul, H.Z. The relationship between neutrophil-to-lymphocyte ratio and inflammation in end-stage renal disease patients. *Ren. Fail.* **2012**, *34*, 155–159. [CrossRef]
44. Malhotra, R.; Marcelli, D.; von Gersdorff, G.; Grassmann, A.; Schaller, M.; Bayh, I.; Scatizzi, L.; Etter, M.; Guinsburg, A.; Barth, C.; et al. Relationship of neutrophil-to-lymphocyte ratio and serum albumin levels with C-reactive protein in hemodialysis patients: Results from two international cohort studies. *Nephron* **2015**, *130*, 263–270. [CrossRef] [PubMed]
45. Li, H.; Lu, X.; Xiong, R.; Wang, S. High neutrophil-to-lymphocyte ratio predicts cardiovascular mortality in chronic hemodialysis patients. *Mediat. Inflamm.* **2017**, *2017*, 9327136. [CrossRef]
46. Erdem, E.; Coşkun, K.A.; Karatas, A.; Dilek, M.; Akpolat, T. Neutrophil to lymphocyte ratio in predicting short-term mortality in hemodialysis patients. *J. Exp. Clin.* **2013**, *30*, 129–132. [CrossRef]
47. Amsterdam, E.A.; Wenger, N.K.; Brindis, R.G.; Casey, D.E., Jr.; Ganiats, T.G.; Holmes, D.R., Jr.; Jaffe, A.S.; Jneid, H.; Kelly, R.F.; Kontos, M.C.; et al. 2014 AHA/ACC guideline for the management of patients with non-ST-elevation acute coronary syndromes: Executive summary: A report of the American College of Cardiology/American Heart Association Task Force on Practice Guidelines. *Circulation* **2014**, *130*, 2354–2394. [CrossRef]
48. O'Gara, P.T.; Kushner, F.G.; Ascheim, D.D.; Casey, D.E., Jr.; Chung, M.K.; de Lemos, J.A.; Ettinger, S.; Fang, J.C.; Fesmire, F.M.; Franklin, B.A.; et al. 2013 ACCF/AHA guideline for the management of ST-elevation myocardial infarction: Executive summary: A report of the American College of Cardiology Foundation/American Heart Association Task Force on Practice Guidelines. *Circulation* **2013**, *127*, 529–555. [CrossRef]

medicina

MDPI

Article

Intra-Cranial Arterial Calcifications in Hemodialysis Patients

Feda Fanadka [1], Ilan Rozenberg [2,3,*,†], Naomi Nacasch [2,3], Yael Einbinder [2,3], Sydney Benchetrit [2,3], Ori Wand [4], Tammy Hod [3,5] and Keren Cohen-Hagai [2,3,*,†]

1 Department of Radiology, Meir Medical Center, Kfar Saba 4428164, Israel; feda.fanadka@clalit.org.il
2 Department of Nephrology and Hypertension, Meir Medical Center, Kfar Saba 4428164, Israel
3 Faculty of Medicine, Tel Aviv University, Tel Aviv 6997801, Israel
4 Pulmonary Division, Barzilai Medical Center, Ashkelon 7830604, Israel
5 Department of Nephrology and Hypertension, Sheba Medical Center, Ramat Gan 5262000, Israel
* Correspondence: ilan.rozenberg@clalit.org.il (I.R.); keren.cohen@clalit.org.il (K.C.-H.)
† These authors contributed equally to this work.

Abstract: *Background and objectives*: Vascular calcification is an integral part of atherosclerosis and has been reported to be an independent risk factor for cardiovascular diSsease. Intra Cranial Arterial Calcifications (ICAC) in maintenance hemodialysis (MHD) is highly prevalent. *Materials and Methods*: The aim of this retrospective study was to assess the predictors and outcomes of ICAC in MHD patients compared to a control group without kidney disease. A blinded neuroradiologist graded ICAC in brain imaging (computerized tomography) of MHD patients. Age- and sex-matched patients with normal kidney function served as the control group. *Results*: A total of 280 patients were included in the cohort; 140 of them were MHD patients with a mean ICAC score of 2.3 ± 0.2 versus a mean ICAC score of 1.4 ± 0.2 in the control group ($p < 0.01$). More than 90% of hemodialysis patients in our study had some degree of ICAC. Lower albumin and higher phosphorus and CRP levels were associated with increased ICACs. The multivariate analysis model for predictors of 1-year mortality demonstrated an increased odds ratio for mortality as the ICAC score increased. *Conclusions:* ICAC is very prevalent among MHD patients and results not simply from passive deposition of calcium and phosphate but rather from complex and active processes involving inflammation and structural changes in blood vessels. ICAC independently predicted all-cause mortality and may help with risk stratification of this high-risk population.

Keywords: arterial calcification; hemodialysis; end stage kidney disease; atherosclerosis

1. Introduction

Abnormal structural neuroimaging is commonly seen among patients with chronic kidney disease (CKD) and is even more common among patients with end-stage kidney disease (ESKD) on hemodialysis (HD). Several studies have found structural neuroimaging abnormalities such as cerebral atrophy, white matter hyperintensity, small and large vessel infarcts, and intracranial arterial calcifications. The prevalence of all these abnormalities is higher among HD patients than it is among patients without kidney disease [1–4].

Intracranial arterial calcifications (ICAC) are a common finding in neuroimaging of HD patients [5]. Arterial calcification is an integral feature of active atherosclerosis, occurring in up to 90% of atheromatous lesions. It may be used as a non-invasive marker of atherosclerosis because calcium deposits can be easily detected on non-contrast CT. A strong correlation has been demonstrated between coronary calcifications and coronary plaques. Coronary artery calcification score is a sensitive marker for predicting acute coronary disease [6–8].

ICAC is also considered a relatively sensitive and specific marker of intracranial atherosclerosis in the general population. Aging, traditional cardiovascular risk factors, and CKD have been associated with ICAC. Its presence and severity reflect intracranial atherosclerosis, increased risk of ischemic stroke, vascular events, and death in the general population [6–8].

ICAC in HD patients has a prevalence ranging from 76% to 95%, and its severity is correlated with age, hemodialysis vintage, and serum phosphate levels [5,9]. The association between atherosclerosis and calcification has been established in CKD patients, as well as the resultant cardiovascular disease.

Jablonski and Chonchol [10] reviewed the pathophysiology of vascular calcifications in patients with ESRD, which is extensively deposited in the media layer of the vasculature and is associated with increased arterial stiffness that results in increased systolic blood pressure (SBP), reduced diastolic blood pressure (DBP) and consequently, increased pulse pressure (PP). These changes, with their associated increased cardiac afterload, compromise coronary artery perfusion during diastole, and subsequent left ventricular remodeling and hypertrophy are commonly seen. Simultaneously, coronary plaque increases the risk of myocardial infarction and heart failure, and thus, cardiovascular morbidity and mortality [10].

Aim

The current study assessed the predictors of intracranial arterial calcifications in hemodialysis patients compared to a control group without kidney disease. We also assessed the correlation between ICAC and overall mortality among HD patients.

2. Materials and Methods

2.1. Study Design

This retrospective case–control cohort study included chronic HD patients who had undergone brain non-contrast computerized tomography (CT) from 1 January 2015 until 31 December 2017. Brain imaging was performed as part of the routine evaluation and management of the patients (e.g., after a fall or head trauma).

2.2. Calcification Scoring

A neuroradiologist who was blinded to the clinical and laboratory information of the study population performed repeated and directed radiologic assessment of brain CTs and scored the intracranial arterial calcification. Assessment of thickness of the calcifications in the wall of both common carotid arteries using a score from 0 to 4 as follows [11]: 0—No calcifications, 1—Calcification 1 mm thick or stippled, 2—Calcification 2 mm thick, thin continuous, or thick discontinuous, 3—Calcification 3 mm thick, or thick continuous, 4—Calcification of >3 mm thick or double tracts. For analysis, we have categorized those ICAC results into three categories: patients with a score of 0 were classified as low ICAC, scores 1 and 2 were categorized as medium ICAC and scores of 3 and 4 were grouped as high ICAC.

2.3. Study Population and Data Collection

Chronic HD was defined as a minimum of 3 months of dialysis. Most of the dialysis patients were treated using conventional HD schedules (thrice-weekly sessions, 4 hours each) with high-flux membranes. Hypertension in dialysis patients was determined based on a documented diagnosis in the patient's medical record or prescription of antihypertensive medication. Blood pressure measurements were assessed before, during, and after mid-week dialysis sessions and were published and described previously [12]. We included all chronic HD patients who had undergone non-contrast brain CT during the study period. Follow-up for each participant lasted until 31 December 2017 or until the subject died.

Patients with normal kidney function who had undergone brain CT during a visit to the Emergency Department at Meir Medical Center during the study period were matched for age and gender to the HD group and served as the control group. Relevant data were abstracted from the electronic medical records of the HD and control patients. The reason for performing the imaging was not available for all patients and was not adjusted for between the groups. Laboratory data were also collected from the electronic medical records; for HD patients, we collected pre-dialysis laboratory results performed up to 2 weeks prior to the CT, and for controls, we collected results from tests performed on the day of CT.

2.4. Ethical Considerations

The study was approved by the local Institutional Ethics Committee in keeping with the principles of the Declaration of Helsinki. Data were collected anonymously from the electronic medical records without active patient participation.

2.5. Statistical Analysis

Data are presented as numbers and percentages for nominal parameters and as means and standard deviations for continuous parameters. Variables between study groups were compared using ANOVA *t*-test, or chi-square test, according to the scale of measured variables. Correlations were assessed using Spearman and Pearson coefficients of correlation.

A multivariate regression analysis model was constructed to assess 1-year mortality. Model building was performed on the basis of univariate testing and included ICAC as well as other variables, which demonstrated a significant univariate correlation with mortality. Kaplan–Meier survival curves were used to compare mortality over time between groups. p values < 0.05 were considered statistically significant. Data were analyzed with SPSS Version 25 (IBM Corporation, Armonk, NY, USA).

3. Results

A total of 280 patients were included in this study: 140 in the dialysis group and 140 in the matched control group. The mean age of the study cohort was 71 ± 12 years, and 170 (60.7%) were men. Dialysis patients had significantly more traditional cardiovascular risk factors, such as diagnosis of hypertension and diabetes mellitus, and a higher prevalence of cardiovascular disease (peripheral vascular disease, ischemic heart disease, congestive heart failure) than the control group did. Basic demographic data and comorbidities according to ICAC groups are shown in Table 1. The prevalence of hypertension, diabetes mellitus, and atherosclerosis (coronary heart disease and peripheral vascular disease) was higher as the ICAC was higher.

Table 1. Baseline characteristics of patients according to ICAC score (N = 280).

Characteristic	ICAC Score 0 (n = 46)	ICAC Score 1,2 (n = 142)	ICAC Score 3,4 (n = 92)	*p*-Value *
Age, years	57 ± 14	72 ± 10	77 ± 9	<0.01
Male sex	27 (58.7)	90 (63.4)	53 (57.6)	0.65
Dialysis patients	12 (26.1)	63 (44.4)	65 (70.7)	<0.01
Dialysis vintage (months)	30 ± 70	10 ± 13	24 ± 26	0.148
Comorbidities				
Ischemic heart disease	5 (10.9)	37 (26.1)	40 (44.4)	<0.01
Heart failure	3 (6.5)	21 (14.8)	32 (35.2)	<0.01
Atrial Fibrillation	3 (6.5)	20 (14.1)	23 (25.3)	0.01
Prior stroke	10 (21.7)	38 (26.8)	31 (34.1)	0.27
Diabetes mellitus	10 (21.7)	58 (40.8)	59 (64.8)	<0.01
Peripheral vascular disease	1 (2.2)	10 (7.0)	13 (14.3)	0.04
Hypertension	22 (47.8)	108 (76.1)	76 (83.5)	<0.01

Table 1. Cont.

Characteristic	ICAC Score 0 (n = 46)	ICAC Score 1,2 (n = 142)	ICAC Score 3,4 (n = 92)	p-Value *
Chronic medications				
Aspirin	16 (34.8)	72 (50.7)	57 (63.3)	<0.01
Warfarin	1 (2.2)	5 (3.5)	9 (10.0)	0.06
Statins	16 (34.8)	66 (46.5)	47 (52.2)	0.16
Calcium Carbonate	6 (13.0)	24 (16.9)	20 (22.2)	0.38
Non-calcium-based phosphorus binders	3 (6.5)	10 (7.0)	13 (14.1)	0.15
Beta Blockers	10 (21.7)	64 (45.1)	48 (53.3)	<0.01
ACEI/ARB	8 (17.4)	42 (29.6)	32 (35.6)	0.09
Calcium channel blockers	10 (21.7)	40 (28.2)	35 (38.9)	0.08
Laboratory				
Hemoglobin (g/dL)	13.0 ± 1.8	12.0 ± 2.0	10.7 ± 2.0	<0.01
Albumin (gram/dL)	3.3 ± 0.7	3.4 ± 0.6	3.4 ± 0.6	0.6
Creatinine (mg/dL)	3.8 ± 12	2.9 ± 2.5	4.1 ± 2.6	0.2
Total calcium (mg/dL)	8.8 ± 0.9	8.9 ± 0.9	8.5 ± 0.8	0.04
Phosphorus (mg/dL)	4.1 ± 1.7	4.5 ± 2	5.2 ± 1.6	0.005
Calcium phosphorus product	35 ± 12	39 ± 16	44 ± 13	0.006
PTH (pg/mL)	268± 251	308 ± 187	314 ± 178	0.8
C reactive protein (mg/dL)	6.3 ± 9	6.6 ± 10	4.8 ± 6.7	0.3

ACEI, angiotensin-converting enzyme inhibitor; ARB, angiotensin II receptor blockers; PTH, parathyroid hormone.
* Presented p-values represent the difference between the 3 ICAC categories.

The distribution of ICAC in the study population is shown in Figure 1. Mean ICAC was significantly higher in HD patients than in controls, 2.3 ± 1.3 vs. 1.4 ± 1.1, respectively ($p < 0.01$, Figure 1). A total of 24.3% of the control group did not have any calcifications on CT, as compared with only 8.6% in the dialysis group.

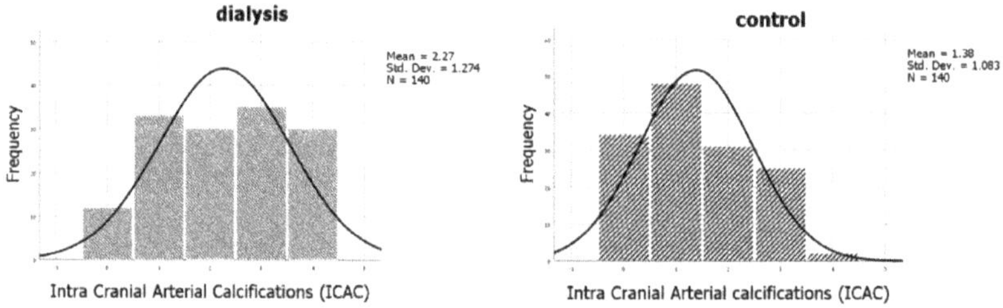

Figure 1. Distribution of intra-cranial calcifications among the study population.

Comparison of the distribution of intracranial calcifications in dialysis versus the control group revealed a significantly different distribution, $p < 0.01$. Mean intra-cranial calcifications were 2.27 ± 1.27 in dialysis patients vs. 1.38 ± 1.08 in the control group, $p < 0.01$.

There was a trend toward increased prevalence of chronic Warfarin treatment with increasing severity of ICAC in the entire study population ($p = 0.06$), as well as in the subgroup of HD patients. Chronic Warfarin use among dialysis patients was higher in patients with ICAC = 1 or 2 (12.7%), as compared with those with ICAC = 0 (4%), $p = 0.06$, OR 3.5 (0.89–13.7). Mean ICAC was 2.64 ± 1.1 in dialysis patients treated with Warfarin and 2.25 ± 1.3 in dialysis patients that were not treated using Warfarin ($p = 0.336$).

We found significant positive correlations between age and ICAC among dialysis patients and the control group. The dialysis group had more ICAC at younger ages than the control group (Figure 2).

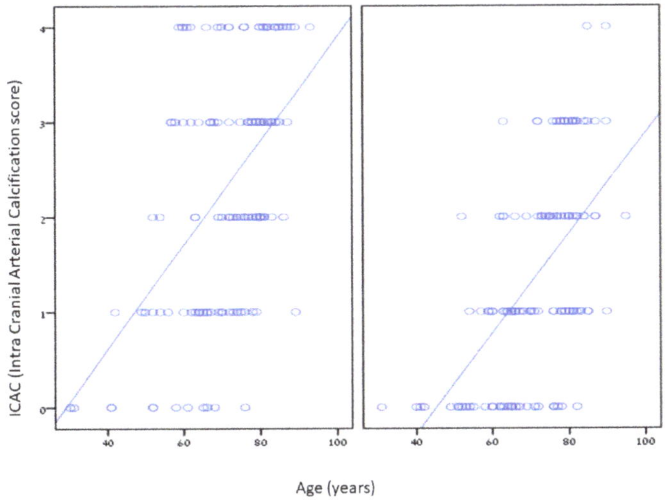

Figure 2. Intra Cranial Arterial calcifications (ICAC) as a function of age. (**Left**): correlation between age and intracranial calcifications (ICAC) score in dialysis patients; (**Right**): control patients. $p < 0.01$.

Dialysis vintage did not correlate significantly with ICAC.

Serum phosphorus levels were positively correlated to ICAC in the dialysis group (mean serum Phosphorus 5.5 ± 1.9 mg/dL, $p = 0.02$) but not in the control group (mean serum Phosphorus 3.3 ± 0.6 mg/dL, $p = 0.929$). Calcium and PTH levels did not correlate with ICAC in either group (mean total calcium level 8.4 ± 0.9 mg/dL in dialysis and 9.3 ± 0.8 in the control group, $p = 0.852$, mean PTH level 309 ± 190 pg/mL in dialysis patients, $p = 0.175$). Albumin and CRP were correlated with ICAC in the dialysis group ($p = 0.001$, 0.007, respectively; albumin was inversely correlated with ICAC).

Mortality rates over time were higher among dialysis patients with higher ICAC. This remained significant even after adjusting for age and comorbidities. The survival curve of dialysis patients according to ICAC score is shown in Figure 3. The multivariate analysis model for predictors of 1-year mortality showed a significantly higher risk for mortality with increased ICAC (Table 2). Heart failure and ischemic heart disease were also significant predictors of 1-year mortality in the multivariate model.

Table 2. Multivariate analysis model for predictors of 1-year mortality among HD patients.

Coefficients	Odds Ratio	95% Confidence Interval Lower	95% Confidence Interval Upper	*p* Value
ICAC = 0		Reference		
ICAC = 1	3	0.6	14.7	0.2
ICAC = 2	9.3	2	44	0.005
ICAC = 3	8.4	1.8	40	0.007
ICAC = 4	8.2	1.6	43	0.01
Hypertension	1.4	0.6	3.3	0.4
Diabetes mellitus	1.0	0.5	2	0.9
Atrial fibrillation	0.7	0.3	1.6	0.4
Congestive heart failure	2.4	1.2	4.9	0.02
Ischemic heart disease	2.4	1.3	4.5	0.006
Peripheral vascular disease	1.6	0.6	4.3	0.3

Intra Cranial Calcification, ICAC.

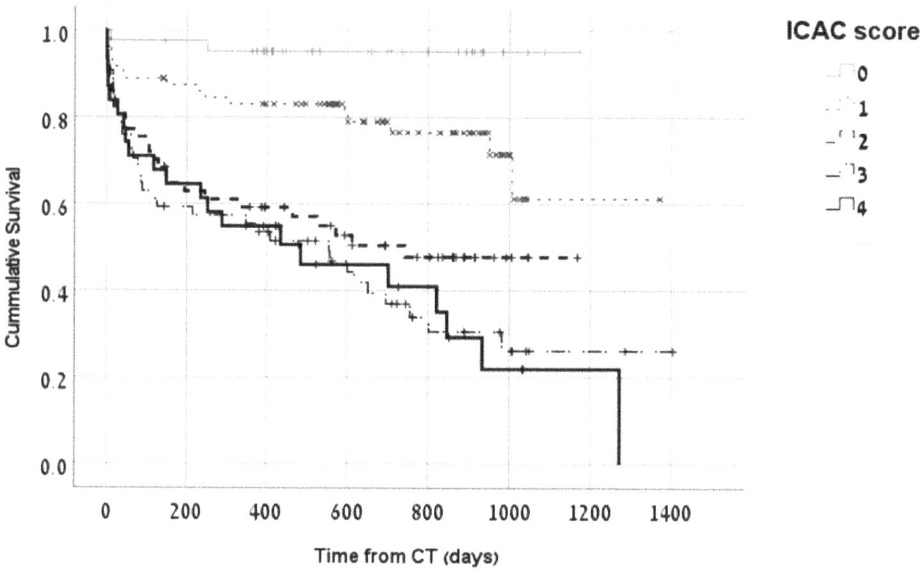

Figure 3. Kaplan–Meier survival curves of dialysis patients according to ICAC. Overall mortality over time was significantly higher for hemodialysis patients with higher ICAC scores, $p < 0.01$.

4. Discussion

ICAC is easily identifiable in simple neuroimaging, such as non-contrast brain CT, which is often performed among dialysis patients. The presence and the severity of vascular calcification can be easily assessed for each patient and may serve as a cardiovascular marker [13]. In this study, we demonstrated that HD patients had a higher prevalence and severity of ICAC compared to a control group. These vascular calcifications also predicted mortality in dialysis patients and were significantly associated with their inflammatory and nutritional status.

More than 90% of hemodialysis patients in our study had some degree of ICAC. As previously described [7,10], ICAC was prevalent among our end-stage kidney disease patients probably since CKD and its associated comorbidities, including mineral bone disorder, are important risk factors for vascular calcifications.

The prevalence of risk factors such as age, diabetes mellitus, and atherosclerotic disease itself, manifested as ischemic heart disease and peripheral vascular disease, increased as the ICAC score increased. ICAC is arterial calcifications that are assumed to be an integral part of active atherosclerosis and were expected to be associated with these variables [6–8].

Although ICAC was higher as the Calcium-phosphorus product increased, we did not find any significant difference in serum levels of total calcium or phosphorus binder medications and ICAC score. There was a positive correlation between ICAC and phosphorus. Although calcium and phosphorus levels are important for the initiation and progression of calcifications, it is well-known that calcification is not a passive deposition of calcium and phosphate but a complex process resulting from many additional variables, and metabolic insults of diabetes, uremia, oxidative stress, and inflammation [10,14,15].

On correlation analysis, we found a significant association between the inflammatory marker CRP and a decrease in albumin as the ICAC score increased. The contribution of inflammation and malnutrition to vascular calcification was described by Choi et al. [14], probably a result of induction of osteogenic phenotype of vascular smooth muscle cells and stimulation of osteoblastic genes by inflammatory cytokines. Systemic inflammation, in both diabetic and non-diabetic environments, aggravates endothelial dysfunction and the atherosclerosis process [16–19].

Active inhibitors of vascular calcification are often down-regulated in patients with ESRD. One of these inhibitors is matrix Gla protein (MGP), a transcription factor that strongly inhibits vascular calcification and requires the activity of a vitamin K-dependent enzyme for carboxylation. Warfarin, a vitamin K antagonist, is assumed to promote vascular calcification via this mechanism [10,20]. In our cohort, 8% of HD patients were treated with Warfarin, and an increasing prevalence of Warfarin use was observed with higher ICAC scores. This increase is interesting and may be related to vitamin K deficiency associated with chronic use of Warfarin. The use of vitamin K antagonists for more than 3 months in adults was associated with a greater burden of intra-cranial calcifications among the elderly population [21].

Vascular calcification can occur in both the intima and media layers of blood vessels, while medial calcification is considered to be more common in patients with CKD, diabetes mellitus, and aging. Medial calcification is associated with increased aortic pulse wave velocity and arterial stiffness [10]. These hemodynamic changes may reduce myocardial perfusion during diastole, especially in the presence of coronary plaques, and lead to increased cardiovascular morbidity and mortality. This explains the increasing mortality as ICAC scores increased, which was reported in other studies, as well [7,8,10,15,22].

The interplay between blood pressure and dialysis is complex and has been extensively investigated. Dialysis patients may have high blood pressure as a result of volume overload, and as seen in our results, hypertension is prevalent among dialysis patients. The dialysis process itself may reduce blood pressure, leading to intradialytic hypotension, which may result in reduced brain blood flow, dialysis-related circulatory stress, regional ischemia, and finally, brain injury. Recently, Intradialytic magnetic resonance imaging (MRI) and spectroscopy demonstrated imaging changes characteristic of cytotoxic edema and ischemic injury [23]. These ischemic intradialytic changes in brain tissue occurred during a single dialysis session, and the coexistence of intracranial vascular calcifications and repeated dialysis sessions with its hemodynamics changes emphasize the importance of additional studies in this field.

In the current study, dialysis vintage did not correlate significantly with ICAC score on brain CT of dialysis patients. This finding is not consistent with other studies and may reflect the multifactorial nature of vascular calcifications and the limitations of the in vivo retrospective design of our study [4,6,7,24]. As mentioned above, vascular calcification is a complex process in disrupted mineral bone disorder, and atherosclerosis initiates a calcification cascade. In our study, ICAC was assessed at only one-time point and by brain CT. As shown by Shroff et al., the calcification process may rapidly progress on dialysis, with a dialysis vintage of even 2 months sufficient to induce histologically overt calcification [24].

The current study had some limitations. First, the study was based on a retrospective, single-center cohort; there might be a selection bias. Second, we did not use the gold standard method for diagnosing brain pathology—magnetic resonance imaging (MRI) because its use is less available in our institution, and we used data from available imaging that was performed to patients according to clinical indications as their physicians decided. The reason for performing the imaging was not available for all patients and was not adjusted between the groups. We do not have data about the FGF23-Klotho axis or specific mineral bone markers that are important players in vascular calcifications.

However, this study has several important clinical implications. We found that intracranial calcifications are very prevalent and severe among dialysis patients and are strongly associated with mortality. The finding of an available and inexpensive prognostic marker, such as ICAC, can help physicians stratify their patients' risk in order to focus on different treatment strategies for higher-risk patients.

5. Conclusions

In conclusion, ICAC is highly prevalent and extensive among dialysis patients. Vascular calcifications do not simply result from passive depositions of calcium and phosphate but rather from complex, active processes involving inflammation and structural changes in blood vessels and hemodynamic changes. These result in increased mortality as the calcification score increases.

Author Contributions: Conceptualization, F.F., S.B. and K.C.-H.; methodology, F.F., N.N. and K.C.-H.; software, I.R.; validation, O.W. and K.C.-H.; formal analysis, K.C.-H.; investigation, Y.E., F.F., S.B. and K.C.-H.; resources, F.F. and N.N.; data curation, F.F. and K.C.-H.; writing—original draft preparation, K.C.-H.; writing—review and editing, F.F., T.H., S.B. and K.C.-H.; visualization, Y.E. and O.W.; supervision, S.B. and K.C.-H.; project administration, F.F. and K.C.-H.; funding acquisition, S.B. All authors have read and agreed to the published version of the manuscript.

Funding: This research received no external funding.

Institutional Review Board Statement: The study was conducted in accordance with the Declaration of Helsinki and approved by the Institutional Review Board of Meir Medical Center (MMC 0251-17, approved in 30 April 2018).

Informed Consent Statement: Patient consent was waived due to the retrospective nature of the study.

Data Availability Statement: The data underlying this article will be shared on reasonable request to the corresponding author.

Acknowledgments: We thank Faye Schreiber for editing the manuscript, Nava Jelin for statistical analysis, and Tania Grumberg for helping collect data.

Conflicts of Interest: The authors declare no conflict of interest.

References

1. Drew, D.A.; Bhadelia, R.; Tighiouart, H.; Novak, V.; Scott, T.M.; Lou, K.V.; Shaffi, K.; Weiner, D.E.; Sarnak, M.J. Anatomic brain disease in hemodialysis patients: A cross-sectional study. *Am. J. Kidney Dis.* **2013**, *61*, 271–278. [CrossRef]
2. Pi, H.-C.; Xu, Y.-F.; Xu, R.; Yang, Z.-K.; Qu, Z.; Chen, Y.-Q.; Liu, G.-L.; Dong, J. Cognitive Impairment and Structural Neuroimaging Abnormalities Among Patients with Chronic Kidney Disease. *Kidney Blood Press. Res.* **2016**, *41*, 986–996. [CrossRef]
3. Savazzi, G.M.; Cusmano, F.; Musini, S. Cerebral imaging changes in patients with chronic renal failure treated conservatively or in hemodialysis. *Nephron* **2001**, *89*, 31–36. [CrossRef]
4. Iwasa, Y.; Otsubo, S.; Nomoto, K.; Yashiro, N.; Yajima, A.; Kimata, N.; Akiba, T.; Nitta, K. Prevalence of intracranial artery calcification in hemodialysis patients—A case-control study. *Int. Urol. Nephrol.* **2012**, *44*, 1223–1228. [CrossRef]
5. Bugnicourt, J.-M.; Chillon, J.-M.; Massy, Z.A.; Canaple, S.; Lamy, C.; Deramond, H.A.A.; Godefroy, O. High prevalence of intracranial artery calcification in stroke patients with CKD: A retrospective study. *Clin. J. Am. Soc. Nephrol.* **2009**, *4*, 284–290. [CrossRef]
6. de Weert, T.; Cakir, H.; Rozie, S.; Cretier, S.; Meijering, E.; Dippel, D.; van der Lugt, A. Intracranial internal carotid artery calcifications: Association with vascular risk factors and ischemic cerebrovascular disease. *Am. J. Neuroradiol.* **2009**, *30*, 177–184. [CrossRef]
7. Wu, X.H.; Chen, X.-Y.; Wang, L.J.; Wong, K.S. Intracranial Artery Calcification and Its Clinical Significance. *J. Clin. Neurol.* **2016**, *12*, 253–261. [CrossRef]
8. Bugnicourt, J.-M.; Leclercq, C.; Chillon, J.-M.; Diouf, M.; Deramond, H.; Canaple, S.; Lamy, C.; Massy, Z.A.; Godefroy, O. Presence of intracranial artery calcification is associated with mortality and vascular events in patients with ischemic stroke after hospital discharge: A cohort study. *Stroke* **2011**, *42*, 3447–3453. [CrossRef]
9. Power, A.; Chan, K.; Haydar, A.; Hamady, M.; Cairns, T.; Taube, D.; Duncan, N. Intracranial arterial calcification is highly prevalent in hemodialysis patients but does not associate with acute ischemic stroke. *Hemodial. Int.* **2011**, *15*, 256–263. [CrossRef]
10. Jablonski, K.L.; Chonchol, M. Vascular calcification in end-stage renal disease. *Hemodial. Int.* **2013**, *17* (Suppl. 1), S17–S21. [CrossRef]
11. Babiarz, L.S.; Yousem, D.M.; Wasserman, B.A.; Wu, C.; Bilker, W.; Beauchamp, N., Jr. Cavernous carotid artery calcification and white matter ischemia. *Am. J. Neuroradiol.* **2003**, *24*, 872–877.
12. Cohen-Hagai, K.; Fanadka, F.; Grumberg, T.; Topaz, G.; Nacasch, N.; Greenberg, M.; Zitman-Gal, T.; Benchetrit, S. Diastolic blood pressure is associated with brain atrophy in hemodialysis patients: A single center case–control study. *Ther. Apher. Dial.* **2022**, *26*, 94–102. [CrossRef]
13. Fanadka, F.; Grumberg, T.; Topaz, G.; Benchetrit, S.; Zitman-Gal, T.; Wand, O.; Cohen-Hagai, K. Intracranial and heart valve calcifications in hemodialysis patients—Interrelationship and clinical impact. *Hemodial. Int.* **2022**, *26*, 527–532. [CrossRef]

14. Choi, S.R.; Lee, Y.-K.; Cho, A.J.; Park, H.C.; Han, C.H.; Choi, M.-J.; Koo, J.-R.; Yoon, J.-W.; Noh, J.W. Malnutrition, inflammation, progression of vascular calcification and survival: Inter-relationships in hemodialysis patients. *PLoS ONE* **2019**, *14*, e0216415. [CrossRef] [PubMed]
15. Mizobuchi, M.; Towler, D.; Slatopolsky, E. Vascular calcification: The killer of patients with chronic kidney disease. *J. Am. Soc. Nephrol.* **2009**, *20*, 1453–1464. [CrossRef]
16. Grant, P.J.; Cosentino, F.; Marx, N. Diabetes and coronary artery disease: Not just a risk factor. *Heart* **2020**, *106*, 1357–1364. [CrossRef]
17. Esser, N.; Legrand-Poels, S.; Piette, J.; Scheen, A.J.; Paquot, N. Inflammation as a link between obesity, metabolic syndrome and type 2 diabetes. *Diabetes Res. Clin. Pract.* **2014**, *105*, 141–150. [CrossRef]
18. Nigro, J.; Osman, N.; Dart, A.M.; Little, P.J. Insulin resistance and atherosclerosis. *Endocr. Rev.* **2006**, *27*, 242–259. [CrossRef]
19. Chopra, S.; Peter, S. Screening for coronary artery disease in patients with type 2 diabetes mellitus: An evidence-based review. *Indian. J. Endocrinol. Metab.* **2012**, *16*, 94–101. [CrossRef] [PubMed]
20. Nigwekar, S.U.; Bloch, D.B.; Nazarian, R.M.; Vermeer, C.; Booth, S.L.; Xu, D.; Thadhani, R.I.; Malhotra, R. Vitamin K-Dependent Carboxylation of Matrix Gla Protein Influences the Risk of Calciphylaxis. *J. Am. Soc. Nephrol.* **2017**, *28*, 1717–1722. [CrossRef]
21. Annweiler, G.; Labriffe, M.; Ménager, P.; Ferland, G.; Brangier, A.; Annweiler, C. Intracranial calcifications under vitamin K antagonists or direct oral anticoagulants: Results from the French VIKING study in older adults. *Maturitas* **2020**, *132*, 35–39. [CrossRef] [PubMed]
22. Topaz, G.; Yehezkel, E.; Benchetrit, S.; Korzets, Z.; Arnson, Y.; Kitay-Cohen, Y.; Pereg, D.; Cohen-Hagai, K. Non-coronary cardiac calcifications and outcomes in patients with heart failure. *J. Cardiol.* **2021**, *77*, 83–87. [CrossRef] [PubMed]
23. Anazodo, U.C.; Wong, D.Y.; Théberge, J.; Dacey, M.; Gomes, J.; Penny, J.D.; van Ginkel, M.; Poirier, S.E.; McIntyre, C.W. Hemodialysis-Related Acute Brain Injury Demonstrated by Application of Intradialytic Magnetic Resonance Imaging and Spectroscopy. *J. Am. Soc. Nephrol.* **2023**, *34*, 1090–1104. [CrossRef] [PubMed]
24. Shroff, R.C.; McNair, R.; Figg, N.; Skepper, J.N.; Schurgers, L.; Gupta, A.; Hiorns, M.; Donald, A.E.; Deanfield, J.; Rees, L.; et al. Dialysis accelerates medial vascular calcification in part by triggering smooth muscle cell apoptosis. *Circulation* **2008**, *118*, 1748–1757. [CrossRef]

medicina

MDPI

Article

Cardiovascular Calcifications Are Correlated with Inflammation in Hemodialysis Patients

Dorin Dragoș [1,2], Delia Timofte [3], Mihai-Teodor Georgescu [1,4,*], Maria-Mirabela Manea [1,5], Ileana Adela Vacaroiu [1,6], Dorin Ionescu [1,7] and Andra-Elena Balcangiu-Stroescu [8]

1 Faculty of Medicine, Carol Davila University of Medicine and Pharmacy, Dionisie Lupu nr 37, Sect 2, 020021 Bucharest, Romania; ileana.vacaroiu@umfcd.ro (I.A.V.)
2 1st Internal Medicine Clinic, University Emergency Hospital Bucharest, Splaiul Independentei nr 169, Sect 5, 050098 Bucharest, Romania
3 Department of Dialysis, University Emergency Hospital Bucharest, Splaiul Independentei nr 168, Sect 5, 050098 Bucharest, Romania
4 Department of Radiotherapy, Prof. Dr. Al. Trestioreanu Institute of Oncology Bucharest, Șos. Fundeni nr 252, Sect 2, 022328 Bucharest, Romania
5 National Institute of Neurology and Cerebrovascular Diseases, Șos. Berceni nr 10–12, Sect 4, 041915 Bucharest, Romania
6 Nephrology and Dialysis Clinic, "Sf. Ioan" Emergency Clinical Hospital, Șos. Vitan-Barzești nr 12, 042122 Bucharest, Romania
7 Nephrology Clinic, University Emergency Hospital, Splaiul Independentei nr 169, Sect 5, 050098 Bucharest, Romania
8 Faculty of Dental Medicine, Carol Davila University of Medicine and Pharmacy, Dionisie Lupu nr 37, Sect 2, 020021 Bucharest, Romania
* Correspondence: mihai.georgescu@umfcd.ro

Abstract: *Background and Objectives*: The main cause of morbidity and mortality in hemodialysis patients is cardiovascular disease, which is quite common. The main objective of our study was to investigate the relationship between oxidative stress, inflammation, and vascular and valvular calcifications in hemodialysis patients. *Materials and Methods*: This observational study had 54 hemodialysis patients, with an average age of 60.46 ± 13.18 years. Cardiovascular ultrasound was used to detect and/or measure aortic and mitral valve calcifications, carotid and femoral atheroma plaques, and common carotid intima-media thickness. The aortic calcification score was determined using a lateral abdomen plain radiograph. The inflammatory, oxidative, metabolic, and dietary statuses, as well as demographic characteristics, were identified. *Results*: There were significant correlations between the levels of IL-6 and carotid plaque number (p = 0.003), fibrinogen level and aortic valve calcifications (p = 0.05), intima-media thickness (p = 0.0007), carotid plaque number (p = 0.035), femoral plaque number (p = 0.00014), and aortic calcifications score (p = 0.0079). Aortic annulus calcifications (p = 0.03) and intima-media thickness (p = 0.038) were adversely linked with TNF-α. Nutrition parameters were negatively correlated with atherosclerosis markers: number of carotid plaques with albumin (p = 0.013), body mass index (p = 0.039), and triglycerides (p = 0.021); number of femoral plaques with phosphorus (0.013), aortic calcifications score with albumin (p = 0.051), intima-media thickness with LDL-cholesterol (p = 0.042). Age and the quantity of carotid plaques, femoral plaques, and aortic calcifications were linked with each other (p = 0.0022, 0.00011, and 0.036, respectively). Aortic annulus calcifications (p = 0.011), aortic valve calcifications (p = 0.023), and mitral valve calcifications (p = 0.018) were all associated with an increased risk of death. *Conclusions*: Imaging measures of atherosclerosis are adversely connected with dietary status and positively correlated with markers of inflammation and risk of mortality.

Keywords: cardiac valve; atherosclerosis; chronic kidney disease; cytokines; interleukin 6; tumor necrosis factor alpha

1. Introduction

The majority of hemodialysis patients have cardiovascular disease, which is the most common complication and the leading cause of death in this population [1,2]. In addition to hemodynamic (primarily volume overload) and metabolic complications of chronic kidney disease (malnutrition, mineral and bone disorders, and anemia), cardiovascular disease is also the most common cause of death in this population [1]. The accelerated calcification of cardiac and vascular structures facilitated by the chronic inflammation typical of these patients plays a key role in the pathophysiological pathways linking CKD to cardiovascular disease, which results in a tenfold increase in cardiovascular mortality among hemodialysis patients compared to the general population [2]. Stenvinkel and colleagues have demonstrated that, in patients on hemodialysis, malnutrition, inflammation, and atherosclerotic cardiovascular disease have an increased prevalence and are independently associated with mortality [3]. As a result, the researchers proposed that all three disorders be combined into a single pathophysiological entity known as "MIA syndrome" [4]. It has since been established that the presence of these problems increases the risk of death in dialysis patients, with the detection of MIA syndrome components being critical in the early identification of these high-risk patients [5]. Atherosclerosis, characterized by the accumulation of lipids and immune cells in arterial walls, stands as a leading cause of cardiovascular diseases, including heart attacks and strokes [6]. Emerging evidence highlights inflammation's critical role in atherogenesis, with TNF-α and IL-6 at the forefront of these investigations [7]. The intricate connection between atherosclerosis markers and pro-inflammatory cytokines, such as tumor necrosis factor-alpha (TNF-α) and interleukin-6 (IL-6), is a complex and highly significant area in cardiovascular research [6]. This issue is crucial because it profoundly impacts our understanding of atherosclerosis development, progression, and potential treatments [7].

This study aims to explore the relationship between vascular and valvular calcifications and the levels of inflammation and oxidative stress in individuals undergoing hemodialysis.

2. Materials and Methods

The present study is an observational study performed on 54 patients (32 males, 22 females, age 60.46 ± 13.18 years) on hemodialysis treatment (for 2–84 months, with an average ± standard deviation of 40.87 ± 22.04 months, with an ultrafiltration of 1.94 ± 0.94 L) in the Hemodialysis Department of the University Emergency Hospital Bucharest, Romania. Eight patients died during the following 6 months, seven from cardiovascular causes and one from bronchopulmonary neoplasm.

Cardiac and vascular ultrasound were used to identify and quantify aortic and mitral valve calcifications and carotid and femoral atheroma plaques (including common carotid intima-media thickness), respectively, while lateral abdominal plain radiograph (in which the spine was visible from the eleventh thoracic to the second sacral vertebra) was employed for the calculation of the aortic calcification score as defined by Kauppila [8].

The biological/biochemical parameters were determined in all 54 patients; radiological assessment was performed in 53 patients (one died before the scheduled radiological examination), while ultrasonographic examination was performed in only 51 patients (the other three died before their turn came for ultrasonographic examination). Ultrasonographic and radiological examinations were performed by certified, experienced specialists blinded to the results of lab tests. The aortic calcification score was derived as an average of the estimations given by two independent examiners, each blinded to the assessment of the other.

Fibrinogen, C-reactive protein (CRP), tumor necrosis factor alpha (TNF-α), interleukin-6 (IL-6), and leucocyte count were used as inflammation markers. As malnutrition markers, we have used biochemical parameters (serum levels of albumin, cholesterol, and triglycerides [9]), dietary intake (normalized protein catabolic rate), and body mass index. As oxidative stress markers we have used total antioxidant capacity, oxalate oxidase 1,

NADPH oxido-reductase, and xanthine oxidase. For fear of missing some important factor, parameters of bone-mineral metabolism (calcium, phosphorus, calcium × phosphorus product, parathormone) and of liver-biliary function (aspartate aminotransferase, alanine aminotransferase, gamma glutamyl transferase, alkaline phosphatase), anemia-related (hemoglobin, ferritin), coagulation-related (platelet count), and hormonal [dehydroepiandrosterone sulfate (DHEAS)] parameters, electrolytes (sodium, potassium), bicarbonate, glycemia, uric acid, and age were also considered.

The study was designed in compliance with the ethical guidelines of the 1975 Declaration of Helsinki. All participants in this study gave their written informed consent. The study was approved by the local ethical committee (Ethical Committee of Emergency University Hospital Bucharest, 6093/31 January 2020).

At first, univariate analysis (UVA) was performed: the correlations between two categorical parameters (such as gender and mitral valve calcifications) were analyzed by means of Fisher's exact test; the correlations between one categorical parameter and one numerical parameter were analyzed by Student's *t*-test (if both sets of numerical values followed a gaussian distribution as assessed by means of Shapiro–Wilk test) or by Mann–Whitney test (if at least one of the two compared sets of numerical values failed to follow a gaussian distribution); the correlations between two numerical parameters were analyzed by computing the correlation coefficient and the associated *t*-statistic (simple regression analysis).

Multivariate analysis (MVA) was then performed, including all the significantly associated parameters (as revealed by UVA) as independent variables.

All the statistical calculations were performed by means of the R language and environment for statistical computing and graphics. The results were considered statistically significant if the *p*-value was below the generally accepted threshold of 0.05.

3. Results

Table 1 is a summary of the demographic, biochemical, and imagistic features of our patients.

Table 1. Anthropometric, biochemical, radiological, and ultrasonographic features of the patients, # patients = number of patients.

Continuous Parameters (Real Numbers)	# Patients	Mean ± Standard Deviation
Body mass index [kg/m2]	54	27.0 ± 5.95
Albumin [g/dL]	54	3.8 ± 0.52
Cholesterol [mg/dL]	54	154.7 ± 41.05
LDL-cholesterol [mg/dL]	54	82.8 ± 27.41
Triglycerides [mg/dL]	54	128.9 ± 72.03
Fibrinogen [mg/dL]	54	383.9 ± 92.92
C-reactive protein [mg/dL]	54	11.6 ± 20.79
Interleukin-6 [pg/mL]	54	27.0 ± 3.2
Tumor necrosis factor-α [pg/mL]	54	14.2 ± 4.21
Cortisol [μg/dL]	54	94.1 ± 135.08
Intima-media thickness [mm]	51	0.6 ± 0.18
Continuous parameters (integer numbers)		Median (1st–3rd quartile) (minimum–maximum)
Aortic calcifications total score	51	3 (0–6) (0–19)
Carotid plaques	51	4 (1–7) (0–>10)

Table 1. *Cont.*

Continuous Parameters (Real Numbers)	# Patients	Mean ± Standard Deviation
Femoral plaques	51	>10 (2–>10) (0–>10)
Categorical parameters (calcifications/plaques)		Present (# patients)/ Absent (# patients)
Carotid plaques	51	42/9
Femoral plaques	51	45/6
Mitral valve calcifications	51	24/27
Aortic annulus calcifications	51	22/29
Aortic valve calcifications	51	25/26
Aortic valve/annulus calcifications	51	31/20
Degenerative aortic stenosis	51	7/44

The vascular access was by tunneled cuffed catheters in 18 patients and by arteriovenous fistula in 36 patients. The primary kidney condition (responsible for the end-stage chronic kidney disease leading to hemodialysis) was: adult type (dominant) polycystic kidney disease (in 5 patients), diabetic nephropathy secondary to type I diabetes mellitus (2), diabetic nephropathy secondary to type II diabetes mellitus (9), focal segmental glomerulosclerosis with nephrotic syndrome (1), IgA nephropathy (1), presumed (not histologically proven) glomerulonephritis (7), congenital renal hypoplasia (1), traumatic or surgical kidney loss (2), drug-induced interstitial nephropathy (1), pyelonephritis due to acquired obstructive uropathy (2), kidney tumor (1), renal vascular disease due to hypertension (21), renal vascular disease due to polyarteritis nodosa (1).

3.1. Associations between Imaging Atherosclerosis Markers and Inflammation-Related Parameters

First, the Shapiro–Wilk test was applied to establish whether the statistically analyzed sets of numerical values followed a gaussian distribution (see Table 2).

Table 2. Results of the Shapiro–Wilk test. A significant (<0.05) p-value (bolded) for at least one of the two sets of numbers indicates that Student's t-test cannot be used and a non-parametric test (such as Mann–Whitney test) should be used instead. Only the pairs of parameters are shown for which subsequently applied tests (Student's t and Mann–Whitney) yielded statistically significant results. TNF-α = tumor necrosis factor alpha; IL-6 = interleukin 6.

Categorical Parameter	Numerical Parameter	Calcifications/Plaques Present		Calcifications/Plaques Absent		Mann–Whitney Test Needed
		Shapiro–Wilk Statistic	p Yielded by Shapiro–Wilk Test	Shapiro–Wilk Statistic	p Yielded by Shapiro–Wilk Test	
Mitral valve calcifications	Cortisol	0.96	0.5	0.96	0.4	No
Aortic valve/annulus calcifications	Fibrinogen	0.89	0.003	0.96	0.5	Yes
Carotid plaques	IL-6	0.96	0.1	0.93	0.5	No
Aortic valve/annulus calcifications	C-reactive protein	0.58	3×10^{-8}	0.6	3×10^{-6}	Yes
Aortic annulus calcifications	TNF-α	0.93	0.1	0.97	0.5	No

Positive statistically significant correlations were found between the presence of aortic valve/annulus calcifications and the level of fibrinogen (see Table 3 and Figure S1), between the presence of carotid plaques and the level of IL-6, and between the presence of aortic annulus calcifications and the level of TNF-α (see Table 4 and Figure S2). However, a surprising negative statistically significant correlation was also found between the presence of mitral valve calcifications and cortisol level (see Table 4 and Figure S2). The correlation between the presence of aortic valve/annulus calcifications and the level of CRP was close to the accepted level of statistical significance (see Table 3 and Figure S1). Regression analysis revealed several other positive associations between various imaging atherosclerosis markers (intima-media thickness, number of carotid plaques, number of femoral plaques, total radiologic score of aortic calcifications) and fibrinogen blood level (see Table 5 and Figure S3). Nonetheless, unexpected negative correlations were found between TNF-α level and aortic annulus calcifications (see Table 4 and Figure S2) and intima-media thickness (see Table 5 and Figure S3).

Table 3. Associations between imaging atherosclerosis markers (aortic valve/annulus calcifications—a categorical parameter) and inflammatory parameters (continuous numerical parameter) assessed by Mann–Whitney test. # patients = number of patients; q1 = 1st quartile 1; q3 = 3rd quartile.

Categorical Parameter	Continuous Parameter	Calcifications Present		Calcifications Absent		W Statistic	*p*-Value
		# Patients	Median (q1–q3)	# Patients	Median (q1–q3)		
Aortic valve/annulus calcifications	Fibrinogen [mg/dL]	31	389 (331.15–437.15)	20	341.5 (315.45–374.2)	410	0.05
Aortic valve/annulus calcifications	C-reactive protein [mg/dL]	31	5.4 (0.7–14.9)	20	1.65 (0.1–6.15)	405	0.07

Table 4. Associations between imaging atherosclerosis markers (aortic valve/annulus calcifications—a categorical parameter) and inflammatory parameters (continuous numerical parameter) assessed by Student's *t*-test. # patients = number of patients; stdDev = standard deviation; TNF-α = tumor necrosis factor alpha; IL-6 = interleukin 6.

Categorical Parameter	Continuous Parameter	Calcifications/Plaques Present		Calcifications/Plaques Absent		*t*-Statistic	*p*-Value
		# Patients	Average ± stdDev	# Patients	Average ± stdDev		
Mitral valve calcifications	Cortisol [mcg/dL]	24	12.67 ± 3.29	27	15.68 ± 4.47	−2.75	0.008
Carotid plaques	IL-6 [pg/mL]	42	7.26 ± 1.05	9	6.41 ± 0.6	3.32	0.003
Aortic annulus calcifications	TNF-α [pg/mL]	22	7.88 ± 0.81	29	8.44 ± 1.02	−2.21	0.03

3.2. Associations between Imaging Atherosclerosis Markers and Metabolic/Nutrition Parameters

Several statistically significant negative associations were discovered between metabolic/nutritional parameters and the majority of imaging atherosclerotic indicators (see Table 6 and Figure S4).

3.3. Associations between Imaging Atherosclerosis Markers and Demographic Parameters

No correlations were found for gender. Nevertheless, age correlated positively with the number of carotid and femoral plaques and the total radiologic score of aortic calcifications (see Table 7 and Figure S5).

Table 5. Associations between imaging atherosclerosis markers (aortic calcifications/mitral calcifications/carotid plaques—the dependent variable) and inflammatory parameters (independent variables) assessed by regression analysis. TNF-α = tumor necrosis factor alpha.

Dependent Variable	Independent Variable	Correlation Coefficient (Confidence Interval)	*t*-Statistic	*p*-Value
Intima-media thickness [mm]	Fibrinogen [mg/dL]	0.46 (0.21–0.65)	3.62	0.0007
Number of carotid plaques	Fibrinogen [mg/dL]	0.3 (0.02–0.53)	2.17	0.035
Number of femoral plaques	Fibrinogen [mg/dL]	0.51 (0.27–0.69)	4.14	0.00014
Aortic calcifications total score	Fibrinogen [mg/dL]	0.36 (0.1–0.58)	2.77	0.0079
Intima-media thickness [mm]	TNF-α [pg/mL]	−0.29 [(−0.52)–(−0.02)]	−2.13	0.038

Table 6. Associations between imaging atherosclerosis markers (total radiologic score of aortic calcifications/carotid plaques/femoral plaques—dependent variables) and metabolic/nutrition parameters (independent variable) assessed by regression analysis.

Dependent Variable	Independent Variable	Correlation Coefficient [(Confidence Interval)]	*t*-Statistic	*p*-Value
Number of carotid plaques	Albumin [g/dL]	−0.34 [(−0.57)–(−0.08)]	−2.56	0.013
Aortic calcifications total score	Albumin [g/dL]	−0.27 [(−0.5)–0]	−2.00	0.051
Number of carotid plaques	Body mass index	−0.29 [(−0.52)–(−0.02)]	−2.13	0.039
Intima-media thickness [mm]	LDL-cholesterol [mg/dL]	−0.29 [(−0.52)–(−0.01)]	−2.09	0.042
Number of carotid plaques	Triglycerides [mg/dL]	−0.32 [(−0.55)–(−0.05)]	−2.38	0.021

Table 7. Associations between imaging atherosclerosis markers (total radiologic score of aortic calcifications/carotid plaques/femoral plaques—dependent variables) and age (independent variable) assessed by regression analysis.

Dependent Variable	Independent Variable	Correlation Coefficient (Confidence Interval)	*t*-Statistic	*p*-Value
Number of carotid plaques	Age [years]	0.42 (0.16–0.62)	3.24	0.0022
Number of femoral plaques	Age [years]	0.51 (0.28–0.69)	4.20	0.00011
Total score	Age [years]	0.29 (0.02–0.52)	2.15	0.036

3.4. Associations between Imaging Atherosclerosis Markers and Other Parameters

No associations were found with the markers of oxidative stress, with the parameters of bone-mineral metabolism and liver-biliary function, with anemia and coagulation-related parameters, with DHEAS, electrolytes, bicarbonate, glycemia, and uric acid. The corresponding results are provided as Supplementary Material.

3.5. Associations between Imaging Atherosclerosis Markers and Cardiovascular Death

The Fisher's exact test indicated connections between cardiovascular death and imaging indicators of atherosclerosis (see Table 8). Simply stated, all deceased patients had calcifications of the aortic valve, annulus, and mitral valve, but only roughly 35–45% of the surviving patients had such calcifications.

Table 8. Results of the Fisher's test for the association between cardiovascular death and imaging atherosclerosis markers (IAM). The columns 2–5 contain the number of patients in the four categories: deceased with positive IAM (D+IAM+), deceased with negative IAM (D+IAM−), surviving with positive IAM (D−IAM+), surviving with negative IAM (D−IAM−).

Imaging Atherosclerosis Marker (IAM)	D+IAM+	D+IAM−	D−IAM+	D−IAM−	*p*-Value	Odds Ratio
Aortic annulus calcifications	5	0	17	29	0.011	Infinite
Aortic valve calcifications	5	0	20	26	0.023	Infinite
Mitral valve calcifications	5	0	19	27	0.018	Infinite

3.6. Multivariate Analysis

The results of MVA are furnished in Table 9. The complete computations are provided as Supplementary Material.

Table 9. Multivariate analysis (MVA). In the second column, there are the factors independently associated with the markers of atherosclerosis in the first column. The third column contains the estimate, which is the average change in the log odds of the dependent variable associated with a one-unit increase in each independent variable (for the dependent variables influenced by at least two independent variables, according to MVA) and Spearman's rank correlation coefficient (for the dependent variables influenced by only one independent variable, according to MVA—namely intima-media thickness and aortic calcifications total score). Spearman's method was used for performing the simple regression analysis as the variables were not normally distributed; no confidence intervals can be calculated by Spearman's method (as it correlates ranks and not actual numbers).

Dependent Variable	Independent Variable	Estimate	95% Confidence Interval	*t*-Statistic	*p*-Value
Carotid plaques	Triglycerides	−0.0022	[−0.0034, −0.00090]	−3.354	0.002
	IL-6	0.13	[0.041, 0.22]	2.845	0.006
Aortic annulus calcifications	Cholesterol	−0.0051	[−0.0081, −0.0021]	−3.374	0.001
	Uric acid	0.12	[0.028, 0.22]	2.536	0.01
Aortic valve calcifications	Age	0.018	[0.0088, 0.027]	3.833	0.0004
	Cholesterol	−0.0030	[−0.006, −0.00005]	−1.993	0.052
Aortic valve/annulus calcifications	Age	0.02	[0.011, 0.028]	4.418	6×10^{-5}
	C-reactive protein	0.0079	[0.0021, 0.014]	2.680	0.01
Intima-media thickness	Fibrinogen	0.3	_	3.62	0.0007
Number of carotid plaques	Age	0.02	[0.011, 0.028]	3.546	0.0009
	BMI	0.0079	[0.0021, 0.014]	−2.518	0.015
Number of femoral plaques	Fibrinogen	0.02	[0.011, 0.028]	3.244	0.002
	Age	0.0079	[0.0021, 0.014]	3.252	0.002
Aortic calcifications total score	Fibrinogen	0.35	_	2.77	0.008

4. Discussion

There is evidence that the amount of atherosclerotic plaques and circulating TNF-α and IL-6 levels are positively correlated, according to numerous studies [10,11]. These results provide credence to the notion that inflammation plays a substantial role in atherosclerosis. Particularly, TNF-α seems to be connected to endothelial dysfunction and the overexpression of adhesion molecules, making it easier for immune cells to be attracted to the vascular wall, which is a critical stage in plaque development [6]. In contrast, research has produced contradictory findings, with some studies suggesting a lack of association or even a negative relationship between the atherosclerotic markers TNF-α, IL-6, and [12,13]. Diverse factors, such as variations in study design, unique patient demographics, and varying measuring procedures, could all contribute to discrepancies between these studies [12]. Additionally, atherosclerosis's temporal element of inflammation adds intricacy [14]. While acute inflammation may exacerbate the formation of plaque, chronic low-grade inflammation may result from atherosclerosis rather than cause it [14]. Atherosclerosis exhibits inherent diversity, manifesting in various phenotypic forms [15]. This diversity could explain some disparities in study outcomes. Additionally, genetic and epigenetic factors modulating the interplay between inflammation and atherosclerosis remain active areas of research [16,17].

In atherosclerosis, the timing and duration of inflammation must be carefully examined. The inflammatory response is dynamic, comprising distinct phases, each potentially affecting plaque stability and progression differently [14]. Therefore, a thorough analysis should consider the specific stage of atherosclerosis under investigation and the markers used to assess disease severity [14].

The therapeutic implications of these findings are significant. If inflammation indeed drives atherosclerosis, targeting TNF-α and IL-6 could be promising strategies to reduce cardiovascular disease risk [6]. Conversely, if chronic inflammation predominantly results from atherosclerosis, interventions focused on lipid management and plaque stabilization may be more relevant [14].

Patients with CKD, especially those in the later stages, make up a subpopulation in which inflammation is quite important. Chronic inflammation causes the vascular endothelium to undergo smooth muscle cell transition and early atherosclerosis development. Through acute-phase proteins such as CRP or cytokines such as TNF-α and IL-6, chronic inflammation greatly contributes to atherosclerosis in both the tunica intima and tunica media layers of the arterial wall [18,19]. According to a recent study [20], TNF-α and IL-6 are key players in vascular calcification because they have a direct impact on smooth muscle cell remodeling at the vascular level and are linked to both intimal and medial calcification. In individuals who are persistently hemodialyzed, IL-6 affects TNF-α's vascular effects and is linked to higher rates of cardiovascular and all-cause mortality [20] Our results showed a positive correlation between imagistic markers of atherosclerosis (intima-media thickness, number of carotid plaques, number of femoral plaques, and aortic calcification score) and plasma fibrinogen level, which is consistent with other researchers' findings of a link between higher fibrinogen levels and carotid intima-media thickness and valvular and vascular calcifications [21,22]. Moreover, it has been displayed that fibrinogen level is higher in patients with carotid atherosclerosis and is positively correlated with intima-media thickness in patients both on hemodialysis and on peritoneal dialysis, with no significant difference between those on hemodialysis and those on peritoneal dialysis [23–25]. Our results demonstrated a statistically significant correlation between aortic valve (both cusps and annulus) calcifications and fibrinogen level, in agreement with the association between high levels of fibrinogen and valvular calcifications demonstrated by other studies [26,27].

On MVA, the association persisted only for intima-media thickness, number of femoral plaques, and aortic calcifications score. For the number of carotid plaques, the association with fibrinogen was effaced by the positive association with age and the negative association with BMI.

Regarding the relationship between CRP and vascular indicators of atherosclerosis in patients with advanced kidney disease, there is no consensus among authors in the literature: Some identified a relationship, while others did not [3,28,29]. Findings from other studies appear to support a synergistic relationship between inflammation and vascular atherosclerosis, which are respectively characterized by higher CRP levels and thicker carotid intima media, in raising cardiovascular and all-cause mortality [30]. In our study,

CRP was associated with aortic valve and annulus calcifications, but the corresponding *p*-value was slightly above the generally accepted level of statistical significance. On MVA, age and C-reactive protein were the factors associated with aortic valve and annulus calcifications. This result matches those already published, suggesting that CRP levels positively correlate with coronary artery calcifications in patients with both early and advanced stages of CKD and that in patients on hemodialysis, CRP is associated with valvular calcifications, with aortic valve calcifications leading to aortic stenosis, with arterial calcification score, and in general with cardiovascular (both valvular and vascular) calcifications [22,27,31–33]. Moreover, CRP has been shown to be an independent predictor of abdominal aortic calcification in patients on both peritoneal dialysis and hemodialysis [34–36].

A higher level of IL-6 was associated with the presence of carotid plaques (at both UVA and MVA) in our patients, which is consistent with the literature, which shows that IL-6 is strongly associated with the severity of carotid atherosclerosis in hemodialysis patients and that increased circulating levels of IL-6 are independently associated with carotid atherosclerosis progression during the first 12 months of dialysis [37,38]. Another study, however, showed that in patients on hemodialysis, the IL-6 level is positively correlated with carotid intima-media thickness but not with the presence of atheroma plaques [37]. The role of IL-6 in the atherosclerotic process was demonstrated in apoE-deficient mice, where recombinant IL-6 injections worsened early atherosclerosis [39]. IL-6 seems to promote atherosclerosis by various metabolic, endocrine, and cellular mechanisms, including increased hepatic synthesis of acute phase reactants, monocyte activation and increased macrophage lipid uptake, lower HDL-cholesterol levels, decreased lipoprotein lipase activity, and activation of the hypothalamic–pituitary–adrenal axis (a potential inducer of obesity, hypertension, and insulin resistance) [40]. IL-6 is involved in the fibrous plaque stage of the atherosclerotic process (Elhage et al., 2001), and high levels of IL-6 are associated with valvular calcifications [26].

Unexpectedly, our findings showed a negative correlation between TNF-α and the occurrence of aortic valve calcifications (cusps and annulus) and carotid intima media thickness. However, the relationships with metabolic variables (uric acid and cholesterol) for aortic annulus calcifications and with fibrinogen for carotid intima media thickness on MVA mask these associations. Some studies have shown a correlation between IL-6 levels and vascular (coronary) calcifications in patients with CKD but not with TNF-α levels; however, other studies have found a significant, albeit weak, correlation between TNF-α levels and the presence of carotid plaques in patients with end-stage renal disease [3,41]. There is a pathophysiological explanation for this association. In vitro studies point out the ability of TNF-α to induce the osteoblastic differentiation of vascular cells and matrix mineralization by calcium incorporation, a process mediated by the protein kinase A-cAMP pathway and resulting in vascular calcification [42].

All 54 patients had their biological and biochemical parameters measured; radiological assessment was performed in 53 patients (one passed away before the scheduled radiological examination), but only 51 patients had their ultrasonograms performed (the other three passed away before their upcoming examination). The association (of both UVA and MVA) between the imagistic markers of atherosclerosis and malnutrition (as reflected by deficient albumin, cholesterol, and triglyceride serum levels, and a lower body mass index) in hemodialysis patients indicated by our results was also demonstrated by other studies [43].

Our findings show a negative relationship between cortisol levels and mitral valve calcification, which contradicts previous findings that cortisol reactivity to stress is associated with the progression of coronary artery calcification and that coronary calcification is associated with a slower decline of cortisol levels throughout the day [44–46]. To our knowledge, there is no information in the literature regarding a putative relationship between cortisol and valvular (either mitral or aortic) calcification.

Age was typically the most highly correlated independent factor on MVA, followed by inflammatory markers (fibrinogen or C-reactive protein) and metabolic (malnutrition-related) parameters (cholesterol or BMI), as was expected for the majority of atherosclerosis markers.

The imagistic markers of atherosclerosis were connected to cardiovascular death in our patients. Aortic valve calcifications (both cusps and annulus) and mitral valve calcifications were seen in all patients who passed away within 6 months, although only 35–45% of the survivors exhibited valvular calcifications. These findings are consistent with recent research showing that patients receiving hemodialysis have a higher chance of dying when their aortic calcification score is above 8 [47,48]. The limitations of our study include the small number of patients enrolled and the time lag between the measurement of biochemical parameters and the imagistic investigation (because performing the ultrasound examination of heart valves and carotid and femoral arteries is laborious and time-consuming).

5. Conclusions

Atherosclerosis imaging markers are positively connected with inflammation markers and risk of death, but adversely correlated with dietary status. More research (ideally larger, multicentric, longer term, and prospective) is required to better clarify the relationship between atherosclerotic lesions and inflammation in CKD patients, particularly those on hemodialysis.

Supplementary Materials: The following supporting information can be downloaded at: https://www.mdpi.com/article/10.3390/medicina59101801/s1, Figure S1: Associations between imaging atherosclerosis markers (aortic valve/annulus calcifications) and inflammatory parameters assessed by Mann–Whitney test; Figure S2: Associations between imaging atherosclerosis markers and inflammatory parameters assessed (y-axis) by Student's t-test; Figure S3: Associations between imaging atherosclerosis markers (y-axis) and inflammatory parameters (x-axis) assessed by regression analysis; Figure S4: Associations between imaging atherosclerosis markers (y-axis) and metabolic/nutrition parameters (x-axis) assessed by regression analysis; Figure S5: Associations between imaging atherosclerosis markers (y-axis) and age (x-axis) assessed by regression analysis.

Author Contributions: Conceptualization, D.D.; data curation, D.T., M.-T.G. and I.A.V.; formal analysis, M.-T.G., D.I. and A.-E.B.-S.; methodology, D.T., M.-M.M., I.A.V., D.I. and A.-E.B.-S.; project administration, D.D.; resources, M.-M.M. and A.-E.B.-S.; software, D.T.; supervision, D.D. and I.A.V.; writing—original draft, M.-M.M. and D.I.; writing—review and editing, M.-T.G. and A.-E.B.-S. All authors have read and agreed to the published version of the manuscript.

Funding: This research received no external funding.

Institutional Review Board Statement: The study was approved by the local ethical committee (Ethical Committee of Emergency University Hospital Bucharest, 6093/31 January 2020.

Informed Consent Statement: The study was designed in compliance with the ethical guidelines of the 1975 Declaration of Helsinki. All participants in this study gave their written informed consent.

Data Availability Statement: The data underlying this article exist as Excel spreadsheets but cannot be shared publicly due to risk of violating the privacy of individuals that participated in the study, as the names of the participating individuals are included in the database. The data can be shared with interested researchers, on reasonable request to the corresponding author.

Conflicts of Interest: The authors declare no conflict of interest.

References

1. Cozzolino, M.; Mangano, M.; Stucchi, A.; Ciceri, P.; Conte, F.; Galassi, A. Cardiovascular disease in dialysis patients. *Nephrol. Dial. Transplant.* **2018**, *33*, iii28–iii34. [CrossRef] [PubMed]
2. Benz, K.; Hilgers, K.-F.; Daniel, C.; Amann, K. Vascular Calcification in Chronic Kidney Disease: The Role of Inflammation. *Int. J. Nephrol.* **2018**, *2018*, 1–7. [CrossRef] [PubMed]
3. Stenvinkel, P.; Heimbürger, O.; Paultre, F.; Diczfalusy, U.; Wang, T.; Berglund, L.; Jogestrand, T. Strong association between malnutrition, inflammation, and atherosclerosis in chronic renal failure. *Kidney Int.* **1999**, *55*, 1899–1911. [CrossRef] [PubMed]
4. Pecoits-Filho, R.; Lindholm, B.; Stenvinkel, P. The malnutrition, inflammation, and atherosclerosis (MIA) syndrome—The heart of the matter. *Nephrol. Dial. Transplant.* **2002**, *17*, 28–31. [CrossRef] [PubMed]

5. Busko, M. MIA Syndrome Strongly Predicts Mortality in Dialysis Patients. *Medscape Intern. Med.* **2006**. Available online: https://www.medscape.com/viewarticle/548026 (accessed on 23 February 2023).
6. Libby, P. Inflammation in atherosclerosis. *Nature* **2022**, *420*, 868–874. [CrossRef] [PubMed]
7. Ross, R. Atherosclerosis-an inflammatory disease. *N. Engl. J. Med.* **1999**, *340*, 115–126. [CrossRef] [PubMed]
8. Kauppila, L.I.; Polak, J.F.; Cupples, L.; Hannan, M.T.; Kiel, D.P.; Wilson, P.W. New indices to classify location, severity and progression of calcific lesions in the abdominal aorta: A 25-year follow-up study. *Atherosclerosis* **1997**, *132*, 245–250. [CrossRef]
9. Zhang, Z.; Pereira, S.L.; Luo, M.; Matheson, E.M. Evaluation of blood biomarkers associated with risk of malnutrition in older adults: A systematic review and meta-analysis. *Nutrients* **2017**, *9*, 829. [CrossRef]
10. Ridker, P.M.; Hennekens, C.H.; Buring, J.E.; Rifai, N. C-reactive protein and other markers of inflammation in the prediction of cardiovascular disease in women. *N. Engl. J. Med.* **2000**, *342*, 836–843. [CrossRef]
11. Danesh, J.; Wheeler, J.G.; Hirschfield, G.M.; Eda, S.; Eiriksdottir, G.; Rumley, A.; Lowe, G.D.; Pepys, M.B.; Gudnason, V. C-reactive protein and other circulating markers of inflammation in the prediction of coronary heart disease. *N. Engl. J. Med.* **2004**, *350*, 1387–1397. [CrossRef]
12. Weiss, T.W.; Arnesen, H.; Seljeflot, I. Components of the interleukin-6 transsignalling system are associated with the metabolic syndrome, endothelial dysfunction and arterial stiffness. *Metab. Clin. Exp.* **2013**, *62*, 1008–1013. [CrossRef] [PubMed]
13. Tzoulaki, I.; Murray, G.D.; Lee, A.J.; Rumley, A.; Lowe, G.D.; Fowkes, F.G. Inflammatory, haemostatic, and rheological markers for incident peripheral arterial disease: Edinburgh Artery Study. *Eur. Heart J.* **2007**, *28*, 354–362. [CrossRef] [PubMed]
14. Tedgui, A.; Mallat, Z. Cytokines in atherosclerosis: Pathogenic and regulatory pathways. *Physiol. Rev.* **2006**, *86*, 515–581. [CrossRef] [PubMed]
15. Virmani, R.; Kolodgie, F.D.; Burke, A.P.; Farb, A.; Schwartz, S.M. Lessons from sudden coronary death: A comprehensive morphological classification scheme for atherosclerotic lesions. *Arterioscler. Thromb. Vasc. Biol.* **2000**, *20*, 1262–1275. [CrossRef]
16. Assimes, T.L.; Roberts, R. Genetics: Implications for Prevention and Management of Coronary Artery Disease. *J. Am. Coll. Cardiol.* **2016**, *68*, 2797–2818. [CrossRef] [PubMed]
17. Shirodkar, A.V.; Marsden, P.A. Epigenetics in cardiovascular disease. *Curr. Opin. Cardiol.* **2011**, *26*, 209–215. [CrossRef] [PubMed]
18. Wang, Y.; Gao, L. Inflammation and Cardiovascular Disease Associated With Hemodialysis for End-Stage Renal Disease. *Front. Pharmacol.* **2022**, *13*, 800950. [CrossRef]
19. Hénaut, L.; Massy, Z.A. New insights into the key role of interleukin 6 in vascular calcification of chronic kidney disease. *Nephrol. Dial. Transplant.* **2018**, *33*, 543–548. [CrossRef]
20. Murt, A.; Yalin, S.F.; Konukoglu, D.; Ronco, C.; Altiparmak, M.R. Fluctuations in Interleukin-6 Levels during Hemodialysis Sessions with Medium Cutoff Membranes: An Analysis on COVID-19 Case Series. *Blood Purif.* **2022**, *51*, 953–958. [CrossRef]
21. Zimmermann, J.; Herrlinger, S.; Pruy, A.; Metzger, T.; Wanner, C. Inflammation enhances cardiovascular risk and mortality in hemodialysis patients. *Kidney Int.* **1999**, *55*, 648–658. [CrossRef]
22. Buyukhatipoglu, H.; Tiryaki, O.; Tahta, K.; Usalan, C. Inflammation as a risk factor for carotid intimal-medial thickening, a measure of subclinical atherosclerosis in haemodialysis patients: The role of chlamydia and cytomegalovirus infection. *Nephrology* **2007**, *12*, 25–32. [CrossRef] [PubMed]
23. Cozzolino, M.; Galassi, A.; Biondi, M.L.; Turri, O.; Papagni, S.; Mongelli, N.; Civita, L.; Gallieni, M.; Brancaccio, D. Serum Fetuin-A Levels Link Inflammation and Cardiovascular Calcification in Hemodialysis Patients. *Am. J. Nephrol.* **2006**, *26*, 423–429. [CrossRef] [PubMed]
24. Tseke, P.; Grapsa, E.; Stamatelopoulos, K.; Samouilidou, E.; Protogerou, A.; Papamichael, C.; Laggouranis, A. Atherosclerotic risk factors and carotid stiffness in elderly asymptomatic HD patients. *Int. Urol. Nephrol.* **2007**, *38*, 801–809. [CrossRef] [PubMed]
25. Zeki Tonbul, H.; Demir, M.; Altıntepe, L.; Güney, I.; Yeter, E.; Türk, S.; Yeksan, M.; Yildiz, A. Malnutrition–Inflammation–Atherosclerosis (MIA) Syndrome Components in Hemodialysis and Peritoneal Dialysis Patients. *Ren. Fail.* **2006**, *28*, 287–294. [CrossRef] [PubMed]
26. Harmankaya, O.; Akalin, N.; Akay, H.; Okuturlar, Y.; Erturk, K.; Kaptanogullari, H.; Kocoglu, H. Comparison of risk factors for cardiovascular disease in hemodialysis and peritoneal dialysis patients. *Clinics* **2015**, *70*, 601–605. [CrossRef]
27. Mohamed, B.A.; Yang, W.; Litt, H.; Rosas, S.E. Valvular calcification, inflammation, and mortality in dialysis patients. *J. Heart Valve Dis.* **2013**, *22*, 584–590. [PubMed]
28. Torun, D.; Sezer, S.; Baltalı, M.; Adam, F.U.; Erdem, A.; Ozdemir, F.N.; Haberal, M. Association of cardiac valve calcification and inflammation in patients on hemodialysis. *Ren. Fail.* **2005**, *27*, 221–226. [CrossRef]
29. Caliskan, Y.; Demirturk, M.; Ozkok, A.; Yelken, B.; Sakaci, T.; Oflaz, H.; Unsal, A.; Yildiz, A. Coronary artery calcification and coronary flow velocity in haemodialysis patients. *Nephrol. Dial. Transplant.* **2010**, *25*, 2685–2690. [CrossRef]
30. Turkmen, K.; Gorgulu, N.; Uysal, M.; Ozkok, A.; Sakaci, T.; Unsal, A.; Yildiz, A. Fetuin-A, inflammation, and coronary artery calcification in hemodialysis patients. *Indian J. Nephrol.* **2011**, *21*, 90–94. [CrossRef]
31. Cao, J.J.; Arnold, A.M.; Manolio, T.A.; Polak, J.F.; Psaty, B.M.; Hirsch, C.H.; Kuller, L.H.; Cushman, M. Association of Carotid Artery Intima-Media Thickness, Plaques, and C-Reactive Protein With Future Cardiovascular Disease and All-Cause Mortality. *Circulation* **2007**, *116*, 32–38. [CrossRef]
32. Stompór, T. Coronary artery calcification in chronic kidney disease: An update. *World J. Cardiol.* **2014**, *6*, 115. [CrossRef]
33. Schönenberger, A.; Winkelspecht, B.; Köhler, H.; Girndt, M. High prevalence of aortic valve alterations in haemodialysis patients is associated with signs of chronic inflammation. *Nephron—Clin. Pract.* **2004**, *96*, c48–c55. [CrossRef] [PubMed]

34. Blacher, J.; Guerin, A.P.; Pannier, B.; Marchais, S.J.; London, G.M. Arterial Calcifications, Arterial Stiffness, and Cardiovascular Risk in End-Stage Renal Disease. *Hypertension* **2001**, *38*, 938–942. [CrossRef]
35. Huang, J.-W.; Lien, Y.-C.; Yang, C.-Y.; Liu, K.-L.; Yen, C.-J.; Wu, C.-K.; Lee, J.-K.; Ho, S.-R.; Wu, H.-Y.; Chiang, C.-K.; et al. Osteoprotegerin, inflammation and dyslipidemia are associated with abdominal aortic calcification in non-diabetic patients on peritoneal dialysis. *Nutr. Metab. Cardiovasc. Dis.* **2014**, *24*, 236–242. [CrossRef] [PubMed]
36. Dhakshinamoorthy, J.; Elumalai, R.P.; Dev, B.; Hemamalini, A.; Sai, P.V.; Periasamy, S. Assessment of abdominal aortic calcification in predialysis chronic kidney disease and maintenance hemodialysis patients. *Saudi J. Kidney Dis. Transpl.* **2017**, *28*, 1338–1348. [CrossRef]
37. NasrAllah, M.M.; El-Shehaby, A.R.; Osman, N.A.; Fayad, T.; Nassef, A.; Salem, M.M.; El Din, U.A.S. The Association between Fibroblast Growth Factor-23 and Vascular Calcification Is Mitigated by Inflammation Markers. *Nephron Extra* **2013**, *3*, 106–112. [CrossRef] [PubMed]
38. Kato, A.; Odamaki, M.; Takita, T.; Maruyama, Y.; Kumagai, H.; Hishida, A. Association between interleukin-6 and carotid atherosclerosis in hemodialysis patients. *Kidney Int.* **2002**, *61*, 1143–1152. [CrossRef]
39. Stenvinkel, P.; Heimbürger, O.; Jogestrand, T. Elevated interleukin-6 predicts progressive carotid artery atherosclerosis in dialysis patients: Association with *Chlamydia pneumoniae* seropositivity. *Am. J. Kidney Dis.* **2002**, *39*, 274–282. [CrossRef]
40. Huber, S.A.; Sakkinen, P.; Conze, D.; Hardin, N.; Tracy, R. Interleukin-6 exacerbates early atherosclerosis in mice. *Arterioscler. Thromb. Vasc. Biol.* **1999**, *19*, 2364–2367. [CrossRef]
41. Yudkin, J.S.; Kumari, M.; Humphries, S.E.; Mohamed-Ali, V. Inflammation, obesity, stress and coronary heart disease: Is interleukin-6 the link? *Atherosclerosis* **2000**, *148*, 209–214. [CrossRef]
42. Kamińska, J.; Stopiński, M.; Mucha, K.; Jędrzejczak, A.; Gołębiowski, M.; Niewczas, M.A.; Pączek, L.; Foroncewicz, B. IL 6 but not TNF is linked to coronary artery calcification in patients with chronic kidney disease. *Cytokine* **2019**, *120*, 9–14. [CrossRef] [PubMed]
43. Tintut, Y.; Patel, J.; Parhami, F.; Demer, L.L. Tumor necrosis factor-alpha promotes in vitro calcification of vascular cells via the cAMP pathway. *Circulation* **2000**, *102*, 2636–2642. [CrossRef] [PubMed]
44. Zyga, S.; Christopoulou, G.; Malliarou, M. Malnutrition-inflammation-atherosclerosis syndrome in patients with end-stage renal disease. *J. Ren. Care* **2011**, *37*, 12–15. [CrossRef] [PubMed]
45. Hamer, M.; Endrighi, R.; Venuraju, S.M.; Lahiri, A.; Steptoe, A. Cortisol responses to mental stress and the progression of coronary artery calcification in healthy men and women. *PLoS ONE* **2012**, *7*, e31356. [CrossRef]
46. Seldenrijk, A.; Hamer, M.; Lahiri, A.; Penninx BW, J.H.; Steptoe, A. Psychological distress, cortisol stress response and subclinical coronary calcification. *Psychoneuroendocrinology* **2012**, *37*, 48–55. [CrossRef]
47. Matthews, K.; Schwartz, J.; Cohen, S.; Seeman, T. Diurnal cortisol decline is related to coronary calcification: CARDIA study. *Psychosom. Med.* **2006**, *68*, 657–661. [CrossRef] [PubMed]
48. Kwon, H.Y.; Lee, O.H.; Kim, M.J.; Joo, W.C.; Lee, S.Y.; Kim, M.-J.; Song, J.H.; Lee, S.W. The association between mortality and abdominal aortic calcification and relation between its progression and serum calcium concentration in chronic hemodialysis patients. *Kidney Res. Clin. Pract.* **2014**, *33*, 95–102. [CrossRef]

medicina

MDPI

Article

Serum Endocan Is a Risk Factor for Aortic Stiffness in Patients Undergoing Maintenance Hemodialysis

Tsung-Jui Wu [1,2,3], Chih-Hsien Wang [4,5], Yu-Hsien Lai [4,5], Chiu-Huang Kuo [4,6], Yu-Li Lin [4,5] and Bang-Gee Hsu [2,4,5,*]

1 Division of Nephrology, Department of Medicine, Hualien Armed Forces General Hospital, Hualien 97144, Taiwan; ahreiwu@gmail.com
2 Institute of Medical Sciences, Tzu Chi University, Hualien 97004, Taiwan
3 Division of Nephrology, Department of Internal Medicine, Tri-Service General Hospital, National Defense Medical Center, Taipei 11490, Taiwan
4 Divisions of Nephrology, Hualien Tzu Chi Hospital, Buddhist Tzu Chi Medical Foundation, Hualien 97004, Taiwan; wangch33@gmail.com (C.-H.W.); hsienhsien@gmail.com (Y.-H.L.); hermit.kuo@gmail.com (C.-H.K.); nomo8931126@gmail.com (Y.-L.L.)
5 School of Medicine, Tzu Chi University, Hualien 97004, Taiwan
6 School of Post-Baccalaureate Chinese Medicine, Tzu Chi University, Hualien 97004, Taiwan
* Correspondence: gee.lily@msa.hinet.net

Abstract: *Background and Objectives*: Endocan, secreted from the activated endothelium, is a key player in inflammation, endothelial dysfunction, proliferation of vascular smooth muscle cells, and angiogenesis. We aimed to investigate the link between endocan and aortic stiffness in maintenance hemodialysis (HD) patients. *Materials and Methods*: After recruiting HD patients from a medical center, their baseline characteristics, blood sample, and anthropometry were assessed and recorded. The serum endocan level was determined using an enzyme immunoassay kit, and carotid–femoral pulse wave velocity (cfPWV) measurement was used to evaluate aortic stiffness. *Results*: A total of 122 HD patients were enrolled. Aortic stiffness was diagnosed in 53 patients (43.4%), who were found to be older ($p = 0.007$) and have a higher prevalence of diabetes ($p < 0.001$) and hypertension ($p = 0.030$), higher systolic blood pressure ($p = 0.011$), and higher endocan levels ($p < 0.001$), when compared with their counterparts. On the multivariate logistic regression model, the development of aortic stiffness in patients on chronic HD was found to be associated with endocan [odds ratio (OR): 1.566, 95% confidence interval (CI): 1.224–2.002, $p < 0.001$], age (OR: 1.040, 95% CI: 1.001–1.080, $p = 0.045$), and diabetes (OR: 4.067, 95% CI: 1.532–10.798, $p = 0.005$), after proper adjustment for confounders (adopting diabetes, hypertension, age, systolic blood pressure, and endocan). The area under the receiver operating characteristic curve was 0.713 (95% CI: 0.620–0.806, $p < 0.001$) for predicting aortic stiffness by the serum endocan level, at an optimal cutoff value of 2.68 ng/mL (64.15% sensitivity, 69.57% specificity). Upon multivariate linear regression analysis, logarithmically transformed endocan was proven as an independent predictor of cfPWV ($\beta = 0.405$, adjusted R^2 change = 0.152; $p < 0.001$). *Conclusions*: The serum endocan level positively correlated with cfPWV and was an independent predictor of aortic stiffness in chronic HD patients.

Keywords: aortic stiffness; carotid–femoral pulse wave velocity; diabetes; endocan; hemodialysis; inflammation

1. Introduction

In Taiwan, although the incidence of end-stage renal disease (ESRD) on maintenance dialysis has numerically decreased for three consecutive years, it remains the highest worldwide, with a prevalence of 3839 per million population in 2021 [1]. Similar to the situation in the United States, cardiovascular disease (CVD) remains the major comorbidity at the end life of a patient on dialysis [2]. Currently, consensus on the overall benefit of intensive blood pressure control has been demonstrated in many randomized clinical trials, including the Modification of Diet in Renal Disease, African American Study of Kidney Disease and Hypertension, Action to Control Cardiovascular Risk in Diabetes, Systolic Blood Pressure Intervention Trial, and Strategy of Blood Pressure Intervention in the Elderly Hypertensive Patients [3–6]. However, in a meta-analysis of the aforementioned studies, the beneficial effect was found to be not applicable to patients on maintenance dialysis [7]. In other words, there is a clear unmet need in the clinical care of patients with ESRD.

Aortic stiffness represents increased cardiac workload and is a proven mechanical biomarker for cardiovascular morbidity and mortality in patients with chronic kidney disease (CKD), with or without dialysis [8,9]. The severity of aortic stiffness could be noninvasively quantified by the velocity of pulse pressure transmission along the arterial tree [10]. Although pulse wave velocity is well recognized for its predictive power, limited availability, various devices, and the requirement of a specialist to perform the measurement were the factors that prevented its widespread adoption in clinical practice [11].

Many clinical studies focused on the correlation between the severity of aortic stiffness in patients with ESRD and various serum biomarkers, such as uremic toxin and inflammatory/atherosclerosis markers [12,13]. In the event of vascular inflammation, adipocytes produce both proinflammatory molecules, such as tumor necrosis factor alpha (TNFα), and anti-inflammatory molecules, such as adiponectin, to interfere with the function of monocytes/macrophages and the production of endocan, which was previously known as endothelial cell-specific molecule-1 (ESM1) [14–16]. In 1996, endocan was first identified as a 20 kDa proteoglycan with a limited expression pattern on endothelial cells of the lungs, kidneys, and umbilical cord [17]. Wellner et al. demonstrated that ESM1 formation in adipocytes is induced by protein kinase C, suggesting its central role in regulating inflammatory processes [18]. The diagnostic and prognostic role of endocan has also been extensively investigated and evidenced in the various events of lung inflammation [19]. Muhammad et al. demonstrated that, clinically, even low-grade inflammation was associated with arterial stiffness in a large, prospectively population-based cohort in Sweden [20]. Aortic PWV was also demonstrated to be positively associated with the inflammatory disease duration and white blood cell count in a systemic meta-analysis study [21]. Khalaji et al. further showed that a relatively high endocan level was associated with CVD risk in patients with impaired renal function [22]. This present study investigated the association of the serum endocan level with a mechanical biomarker for aortic stiffness, as measured by the carotid–femoral pulse wave velocity (cfPWV), in patients on maintenance hemodialysis (HD).

2. Materials and Methods

2.1. Participants and Study Design

After the study protocol was approved by the research ethics committee of Hualien Tzu Chi Hospital, Buddhist Tzu Chi Medical Foundation (IRB109-121-C), patients > 20 years old and on thrice weekly maintenance 4 h standard HD for >6 months at a medical center in eastern Taiwan from 1 July 2021 to 30 September 2021 were screened for this study. The exclusion criteria were malignancy, cerebrovascular accident, acute infection, limb amputation, heart failure, liver cirrhosis, chronic obstructive lung disease, and immobilization. A total of 122 patients on HD were included and provided signed informed consent. Figure 1 depicts the flow chart of this study. The medical records were reviewed for the etiology of renal failure. The diagnoses of diabetes mellitus (DM) and hypertension were confirmed based on the documentation or prescription of antidiabetic or antihypertensive agents. Furthermore, the use of renin–angiotensin system blockers, beta blockers, calcium channel blockers, statins, and fibrates was specifically recorded. This study was conducted following the ethical guidelines of the Declaration of Helsinki.

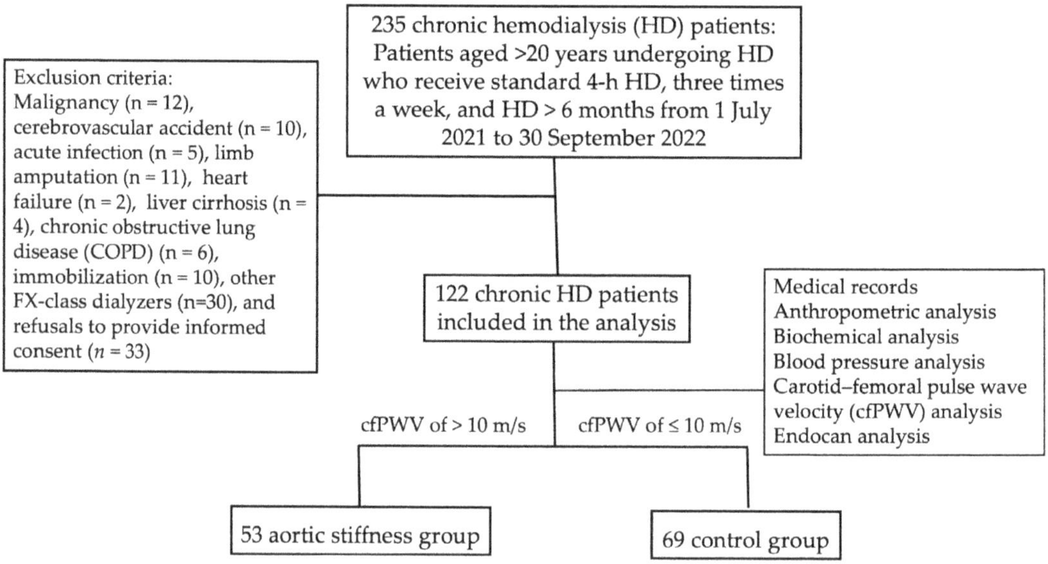

Figure 1. Flow chart of this study.

2.2. *Anthropometric Analyses and Biochemical Investigations*

Blood pressure was taken before the HD sessions after a 10 min seated rest. The body mass index was calculated by dividing the body weight (in kg) measured after HD by the body height (in m^2). Upon HD initiation, approximately 5 mL of blood was drawn from each participant. Once the hemoglobin concentration was determined (Sysmex SP-1000i, Sysmex American, Mundelein, IL, USA), the rest of the blood sample was immediately processed by centrifugation at 3000× *g* for 10 min. For biochemical analyses, the levels of blood urea nitrogen, creatinine, total cholesterol, triglyceride, glucose, albumin, calcium, and inorganic phosphorus were measured by an autoanalyzer (SiemensAdvia 1800, Siemens Healthcare GmbH, Henkestr, Germany). All HD sessions were performed using high-flux polysulfone and non-reused dialyzers (FX class dialyzer; Fresenius Medical Care, Bad Homburg, Germany). The adequacy of HD was determined by urea clearance (Kt/V), using the single pool urea kinetic modeling. The serum levels of endocan (Aviscera Bioscience, Inc., Santa Clara, CA, USA) and intact parathyroid hormone (iPTH) (Abcam, Cambridge, MA, USA) were measured using commercially available enzyme-linked immunosorbent assay kits [12,13].

2.3. *Assessments of Aortic Stiffness by Applanation Topometry*

After asking the participant to relax in a supine position for at least 10 min, the cfPWV was measured using transcutaneous SphygmoCor probe (SphygmoCor system, AtCor Medical, Sydney, Australia), which simultaneously recorded the pulse waveform in the target artery area and electrocardiogram (ECG) [12,13]. After obtaining an accurate and reproducible pulse waveform, we recorded at least 12 s of signal or 10 consecutive cardiac cycles. The arterial path length required for pulse wave velocity calculation was obtained by subtracting the carotid length from the distance between the suprasternal notch and the femoral recording site. Each set of pulse waveforms and ECG recordings were entered into the SphygmoCor software 1.30 (AtCor Medical) for an integrated calculation of the average time difference between the ECG R waves and the pulse waveforms of the two recording sites on a beat-to-beat basis. Thereafter, the cfPWV was automatically generated by the software as the arterial path length divided by the travel time of the pulse wave between two sites. Measurements with <10% standard deviations were included for analysis, and other quality indices were applied to ensure data uniformity. The participant was classified in the aortic stiffness group if the cfPWV was >10 m/s; this represented an increased cardiovascular risk, according to the consensus of the 2018 European Society of Cardiology clinical practice guidelines on arterial hypertension [23].

2.4. Statistical Analysis

All collected data were first examined for normality using Kolmogorov–Smirnov test. Normally distributed data were expressed as mean ± standard deviation and were compared between the two groups using two-tailed independent Student's *t*-test. Data with nonnormal distribution, such as HD duration, cfPWV, triglyceride, glucose, iPTH, and endocan, were expressed as median (interquartile range) and were compared by the Mann–Whitney U test. To conform to normality, skewness was reduced by common logarithmical transformation. The categorical variables were presented as number (%) and analyzed by the χ^2 test. Variables that were significantly associated with aortic stiffness were examined in the multivariate logistic regression model. The simple linear regression model evaluated the clinical variables that correlated with the cfPWV. Those that were significantly associated with the cfPWV were tested for independence using a multivariate forward stepwise regression model. A receiver operating characteristic (ROC) curve was used to examine the diagnostic performance of serum endocan level in predicting aortic stiffness, and the area under the curve (AUC) was calculated to determine accuracy. Data analyses were performed using the statistical software SPSS for Windows (version 19.0; SPSS Inc., Chicago, IL, USA). Statistical significance was set at a p value of <0.05.

3. Results

3.1. Baseline Characteristics

The demographic and biochemical characteristics of the participants are summarized in Table 1. Patients with increased cfPWV were assigned to the aortic stiffness group, and those with normal cfPWV were assigned to the control group. The 122 participants, in total, comprised 53 (43.4%) in the aortic stiffness group and 69 (56.6%) in the control group. There were no differences between groups in terms of sex, HD duration, anthropometric data, general blood biochemistries, HD adequacy, and use of antihypertensive or lipid-lowering agents. Compared with the control group, the aortic stiffness group was significantly older ($p = 0.007$) and had significantly higher systolic blood pressure (SBP, $p = 0.011$), serum endocan level ($p < 0.001$), and prevalence of diabetes mellitus (DM, $p < 0.001$) and hypertension ($p = 0.030$).

Table 1. Clinical variables of the 122 hemodialysis patients with or without aortic stiffness.

Characteristics	All Patients (n = 122)	Control Group (n = 69)	Aortic Stiffness Group (n = 53)	p Value
Age (years)	63.28 ± 12.26	60.68 ± 13.10	66.66 ± 10.24	0.007 *
Female, n (%)	61 (50.0)	37 (53.6)	24 (45.3)	0.361
HD duration (months)	58.26 (25.53–129.60)	80.76 (21.66–144.00)	53.40 (26.70–85.44)	0.268
Height (cm)	159.97 ± 8.59	159.51 ± 9.04	160.57 ± 8.01	0.502
Pre-HD body weight (kg)	63.60 ± 15.10	62.84 ± 15.48	64.59 ± 14.67	0.528
Post-HD body weight (kg)	61.41 ± 14.72	60.70 ± 15.04	62.33 ± 14.37	0.545
Body mass index (kg/m^2)	24.89 ± 4.91	24.71 ± 5.24	25.12 ± 4.50	0.652
Carotid-femoral PWV (m/s)	9.25 (7.50–12.45)	7.70 (7.00–8.80)	12.90 (11.75–14.90)	<0.001 *
Systolic blood pressure (mmHg)	141.59 ± 24.60	136.67 ± 23.52	148.00 ± 24.71	0.011 *
Diastolic blood pressure (mmHg)	76.01 ± 15.03	75.84 ± 14.64	76.36 ± 15.66	0.851
Hemoglobin (g/dL)	10.47 ± 1.17	10.36 ± 1.26	10.62 ± 1.05	0.229
Albumin (g/dL)	4.16 ± 0.47	4.16 ± 0.47	4.16 ± 0.47	0.995

Table 1. *Cont.*

Characteristics	All Patients (n = 122)	Control Group (n = 69)	Aortic Stiffness Group (n = 53)	p Value
Total cholesterol (mg/dL)	145.58 ± 34.12	149.20 ± 37.95	140.87 ± 28.03	0.182
Triglyceride (mg/dL)	113.00 (86.75–178.00)	109.00 (88.00–193.00)	118.00 (85.00–169.00)	0.916
Glucose (mg/dL)	131.00 (108.50–164.00)	129.00 (103.50–151.00)	132.00 (112.50–179.00)	0.187
Blood urea nitrogen (mg/dL)	60.48 ± 14.77	59.74 ± 13.06	61.45 ± 16.82	0.527
Creatinine (mg/dL)	9.32 ± 2.06	9.44 ± 2.04	9.16 ± 2.09	0.455
Total calcium (mg/dL)	9.03 ± 0.78	8.95 ± 0.75	9.14 ± 0.80	0.185
Phosphorus (mg/dL)	4.65 ± 1.32	4.61 ± 1.33	4.70 ± 1.31	0.718
iPTH (pg/mL)	194.95 (58.50–363.05)	239.30 (94.70–366.20)	141.10 (55.55–357.60)	0.287
Endocan (mg/L)	26.63 (14.59–44.80)	18.35 (10.86–30.42)	32.17 (17.89–53.31)	<0.001 *
Urea reduction rate	0.74 ± 0.04	0.74 ± 0.04	0.73 ± 0.04	0.397
Kt/V (Gotch)	1.35 ± 0.17	1.36 ± 0.18	1.33 ± 0.15	0.332
Diabetes mellitus, n (%)	52 (42.6)	19 (27.5)	33 (62.3)	<0.001 *
Hypertension, n (%)	60 (49.2)	28 (40.6)	32 (60.4)	0.030 *
RAS blocker, n (%)	38 (31.1)	19 (27.5)	19 (35.8)	0.236
Beta-blocker, n (%)	40 (32.8)	21 (30.4)	19 (35.8)	0.528
Calcium channel blocker, n (%)	48 (39.3)	28 (40.6)	20 (37.7)	0.750
Statin, n (%)	26 (21.3)	13 (18.8)	13 (24.5)	0.447
Fibrate, n (%)	27 (22.1)	18 (26.1)	9 (17.0)	0.230

Values of continuous variables were expressed as mean ± standard deviation, analyzed by the t-test; non-normally distributed variables were shown as median (interquartile ranges), analyzed by Mann–Whitney U test; categorical values were presented as number (%), analyzed by the χ^2 test. HD, hemodialysis; Kt/V, fractional clearance index for urea. RAS, renin–angiotensin system. * $p < 0.05$ was considered statistically significant.

3.2. Serum Endocan Level and Development of Aortic Stiffness

Table 2 shows the relationships between the clinical variables and aortic stiffness. After proper adjustments for confounding factors (including DM, hypertension, age, SBP, and endocan), the development of aortic stiffness was associated with the endocan level [odds ratio (OR): 1.566; 95% confidence interval (CI): 1.224–2.002, $p < 0.001$], age (OR: 1.040, 95% CI: 1.001–1.080, $p = 0.045$), and DM (OR: 4.067, 95% CI: 1.532–10.798, $p = 0.005$). The relationships between cfPWV and each risk factor were also demonstrated in scattered bar plots (for DM, Figure S1) or regression plots (for age, SBP, and log-endocan, Figure S2).

Table 2. Multivariate logistic regression analysis of the clinical variables related to aortic stiffness among the 122 hemodialysis patients.

Variables	Odds Ratio	95% Confidence Interval	p Value
Endocan, 1 ng/mL	1.566	1.224–2.002	<0.001 *
Age, 1 year	1.040	1.001–1.080	0.045 *
Diabetes mellitus, present	4.067	1.532–10.798	0.005 *
Systolic blood pressure, 1 mmHg	1.013	0.985–1.041	0.368
Hypertension, present	1.309	0.406–4.218	0.652

Analysis of data was done using the multivariate logistic regression analysis (adopted factors: diabetes mellitus, hypertension, age, systolic blood pressure, and endocan). * $p < 0.05$ was considered statistically significant.

In the ROC curve, we demonstrated the diagnostic performance of the serum endocan level for aortic stiffness, with a decent AUC of 0.713 (95% CI: 0.620–0.806, $p < 0.001$) at an optimal cutoff value of 2.68 ng/mL, with 64.15% sensitivity, 69.57% specificity, 61.82% positive predictive value, and 71.64% negative predictive value (Figure 2).

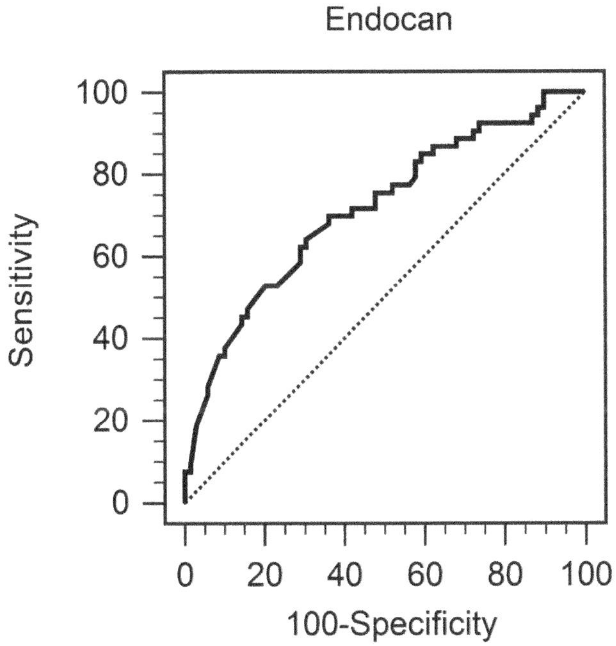

Figure 2. The receiver operating characteristic (ROC) curve of serum endocan level on diagnosing aortic stiffness in the 122 hemodialysis patients. The area under curve (AUC) was 0.713 (95% CI: 0.620–0.806; $p < 0.001$) at an optimal cutoff value of 2.68 ng/mL, with 64.15% sensitivity, 69.57% specificity, 61.82% positive predictive value, and 71.64% negative predictive value.

3.3. Correlations between cfPWV and Clinical Variables

Table 3 shows the correlations between the cfPWV and clinical variables. The cfPWV was positively correlated with age ($r = 0.198$, $p = 0.029$); systolic blood pressure ($r = 0.264$, $p = 0.003$); logarithmically transformed endocan (log-endocan, $r = 0.399$, $p < 0.001$); and the presence of DM ($r = 0.376$, $p < 0.001$). Furthermore, the stepwise multivariate regression analysis showed that the log-endocan level ($\beta = 0.405$, adjusted R^2 change = 0.152, $p < 0.001$) and DM status ($\beta = 0.381$, adjusted R^2 change = 0.141, $p < 0.001$) were the independent predictors of the cfPWV in patients on HD.

Table 3. Correlations between carotid–femoral pulse wave velocity values and clinical variables.

Variables	Carotid-Femoral Pulse Wave Velocity				
	Uni-Variable Regression		Multi-Variable Regression		
	r	*p* Value	Beta	Adjusted R^2 Change	*p* Value
Female	−0.141	0.120	–	–	–
Diabetes mellitus	0.376	<0.001 *	0.381	0.141	<0.001 *
Hypertension	0.170	0.061	–	–	–
Age (years)	0.198	0.029 *	–	–	–
Log-HD duration (months)	−0.135	0.139	–	–	–
Height (cm)	0.112	0.221	–	–	–
Pre-HD body weight (kg)	0.101	0.269	–	–	–
Post-HD body weight (kg)	0.097	0.287	–	–	–
Body mass index (Kg/m^2)	0.067	0.462	–	–	–

Table 3. *Cont.*

Variables	Carotid-Femoral Pulse Wave Velocity				
	Uni-Variable Regression		Multi-Variable Regression		
	r	*p* Value	Beta	Adjusted R^2 Change	*p* Value
Systolic blood pressure (mmHg)	0.264	0.003 *	–	–	–
Diastolic blood pressure (mmHg)	0.079	0.387	–	–	–
Hemoglobin (g/dL)	0.145	0.111	–	–	–
Albumin (g/dL)	0.066	0.473	–	–	–
Total cholesterol (mg/dL)	−0.077	0.399	–	–	–
Log-Triglyceride (mg/dL)	0.056	0.543	–	–	–
Log-Glucose (mg/dL)	0.165	0.070	–	–	–
Blood urea nitrogen (mg/dL)	0.095	0.296	–	–	–
Creatinine (mg/dL)	−0.006	0.947	–	–	–
Total calcium (mg/dL)	0.070	0.440	–	–	–
Phosphorus (mg/dL)	0.070	0.440	–	–	–
Log-iPTH (pg/mL)	−0.103	0.259	–	–	–
Log-Endocan (ng/mL)	0.399	<0.001 *	0.405	0.152	<0.001 *
Urea reduction rate	−0.073	0.425	–	–	–
Kt/V (Gotch)	−0.081	0.377	–	–	–

Data including HD duration, triglyceride, glucose, iPTH, and endocan levels showed skewed distribution and were log-transformed before analysis. Analysis was performed using univariate linear regression and multivariate stepwise linear regression analyses (adopted factors: diabetes mellitus, age, systolic blood pressure, and endocan). HD, hemodialysis; iPTH, intact parathyroid hormone; Kt/V, fractional clearance index for urea. * $p < 0.05$ was considered statistically significant.

4. Discussion

In this study, we demonstrated that among patients on maintenance HD, those who had aortic stiffness were relatively older and had a relatively high prevalence of DM and hypertension, systolic blood pressure, and endocan levels. The odds ratio for aortic stiffness increased by 56.6% with each 1 ng/mL increase in the serum endocan level. Moreover, the serum endocan level exerted a decent predictive performance for aortic stiffness and was independently positively correlated with the cfPWV.

In patients on HD, sodium accumulation from the diet and the lack of self-regulating body fluid homeostasis result in hypervolemia. Consequently, stiffness and remodeling of the left ventricle develop and progress to heart failure [24–26]. In addition to several factors, such as increased systemic sympathetic tone and vascular resistance, inflammation, reduced renal toxin excretion, maladaptation of metabolic/hormonal processes [27,28], arterial stiffness appeared to contribute to the accelerated vascular aging in uremia. Overactivation of the renin–angiotensin–aldosterone system results from the rapid shift of salt and extracellular volume, which is also evident during increased renin activity and aldosterone levels after an HD session [29,30]. On the other hand, endothelial dysfunction can also be present in apparent CKD, acute kidney injury, and even local exposure to uremic toxins in healthy volunteers [31,32]. In an in vitro experiment on subcutaneous arterial resistance in patients with uremia, Morris et al. concluded that endothelial dysfunction was secondary to impaired nitric oxide (NO) production in uremic vessels [33]. In an animal study, Vaziri et al. successfully demonstrated that NO inactivation resulted from the overproduction of reactive oxygen species in a CKD rat and can be ameliorated by antioxidant treatment with high-dose vitamin E [34].

Endocan is a key proteoglycan that integrates with glycoproteins to form the luminal endothelial surface layer, which forms the blood vessel barrier and senses the mechanical transduction of laminar blood flow shear stress to regulate the NO-mediated signaling pathways that play a central role in maintaining vascular homeostasis [35]. Glycocalyx injury, which results in the release of its components into the bloodstream, can be regarded as an early event in endothelial dysfunction and can be quantified by the endocan level [36]. Circulating endocan at the sites of inflammation regulates major processes, such as cell adhesion, and is even involved in tumor progression. Moreover, accumulating experimental evidence suggests that inflammatory cytokines, such as TNFα, and growth factors with proangiogenic potential (e.g., vascular endothelial growth factor, fibroblast growth factor

2, and hepatocyte growth factor/scatter factor hepatocyte growth factor/scatter factor) were strongly associated with the upregulated expression, synthesis, and/or secretion of endocan from the human endothelium [37].

Several clinical studies have addressed the serum endocan level in patients with various severities of renal impairment. Oka et al. found correlations among the serum endocan level, serum TNFα, and the decline in residual urine volume in patients on peritoneal dialysis [38]. Samouilidou et al. showed that increased endocan levels in patients with CKD might be associated with a decreased level of the antiatherogenic protein paraoxonase 1 [39]. In patients with stage 5 CKD without dialysis, endocan seemed to be associated with the circadian heart rate variability [40]. Furthermore, there have been clinical studies that revealed the association of endocan with worse cardiovascular outcomes in patients on peritoneal dialysis [41] and with cardiovascular events and all-cause mortality in patients on HD [42,43]. In a meta-analysis, the endocan level was found to be higher in patients with CKD than in healthy controls, despite the high heterogeneity, and was also demonstrated as a negative prognostic factor in patients on HD, peritoneal dialysis, and even after renal transplantation [22]. The results of our study supported the abovementioned findings and contributed evidence for the clinical use of endocan for CVD surveillance in patients on maintenance HD.

There were several limitations in our study. The nature of a cross-sectional study from a single center might hamper the generalizability of our findings. Endocan could be affected by various conditions, such as dialysis treatment modality or medications [44,45]. Although we excluded patients with acute stress, such as acute infection, cerebrovascular accident, heart failure, liver cirrhosis, chronic obstructive lung disease, malignancy, or chronic deconditioning, such as limb amputation and immobilization, patients in the prodromal stage of this devastating disease could have been easily overlooked, especially those with relatively immune-compromised status secondary to uremia. Diabetes is strongly associated with arterial stiffness, and vice versa [46]. We analyzed only the impact of the presence of diabetes, without further investigating the disease duration. Future research should tackle these shortcomings by including more participants under different dialysis treatment modalities for further subgroup analyses.

5. Conclusions

This emerging endothelial dysfunction biomarker, the serum endocan level, was demonstrated to positively correlate with the surrogate marker of aortic stiffness in patients on maintenance HD, not only in a dose-dependent manner but also with decent predictive power.

Supplementary Materials: The following supporting information can be downloaded at: https://www.mdpi.com/article/10.3390/medicina60060984/s1, Figure S1: Relationships between carotid-femoral pulse wave velocity (cfPWV) and 122 hemodialysis patients with or without diabetes mellitus. The cfPWV among HD patients with or without DM by mean ± standard deviation and was compared between the two groups using a two-tailed independent Student's *t*-test ($p < 0.001$).; Figure S2: Relationships between carotid-femoral pulse wave velocity (cfPWV) and (a) age, (b) systolic blood pressure, and (c) log-transformed endocan (log-endocan) among 122 hemodialysis patients. Two-dimensional scatter plots of cfPWV values with age, systolic blood pressure, and serum log-endocan level among patients undergoing HD are presented in a to c, respectively.

Author Contributions: Conceptualization, T.-J.W. and B.-G.H.; methodology, T.-J.W. and B.-G.H.; formal analysis, T.-J.W. and B.-G.H.; investigation, C.-H.W., Y.-H.L., C.-H.K., Y.-L.L. and B.-G.H.; data curation, C.-H.W., Y.-H.L., C.-H.K., Y.-L.L. and B.-G.H.; writing—original draft preparation, T.-J.W.; writing—review and editing, T.-J.W. and B.-G.H.; supervision, B.-G.H.; funding acquisition, T.-J.W. and B.-G.H. All authors have read and agreed to the published version of the manuscript.

Funding: This research was funded by Hualien Tzu Chi Hospital, Buddhist Tzu Chi Medical Foundation, Hualien, Taiwan, grant number: TCMF-CP 112-03; and Hualien Armed Forces General Hospital, Hualien, Taiwan, grant number HAFGH-D-112013.

Institutional Review Board Statement: The Research Ethics Committee approved the study protocol, Hualien Tzu Chi Hospital, Buddhist Tzu Chi Medical Foundation (IRB109-121-C and approved on 25 May 2020).

Informed Consent Statement: Informed consent was obtained from all subjects involved in the study.

Data Availability Statement: The dataset used, analyzed, or generated in this research is available from the corresponding author, B.-G.H., upon reasonable request.

Acknowledgments: The authors are grateful to all the participants in our study for their time and cooperation.

Conflicts of Interest: The authors declare no conflicts of interest. The funders had no role in the design of the study; in the collection, analyses, or interpretation of data; in the writing of the manuscript; or in the decision to publish the results.

References

1. Chao, C.T.; Lin, M.Y.; Hsu, C.C.; Lin, M.H.; Chou, C.L.; Hsu, Y.H.; Hwang, S.J.; Wu, M.S.; Wu, M.Y. Summary of the 2023 annual report on kidney disease in Taiwan. *Acta Nephrol.* **2023**, *37*, 173–181.
2. Johansen, K.L.; Chertow, G.M.; Gilbertson, D.T.; Ishani, A.; Israni, A.; Ku, E.; Li, S.; Li, S.; Liu, J.; Obrador, G.T.; et al. US renal data system 2022 annual data report: Epidemiology of kidney disease in the United States. *Am. J. Kidney Dis.* **2023**, *81* (Suppl. S1), A8–A11. [CrossRef] [PubMed]
3. Sica, D.A. The African American study of kidney disease and hypertension (AASK) trial: What more have we learned? *J. Clin. Hypertens.* **2003**, *5*, 159–167. [CrossRef] [PubMed]
4. Wright, J.T., Jr.; Williamson, J.D.; Whelton, P.K.; Snyder, J.K.; Sink, K.M.; Rocco, M.V.; Reboussin, D.M.; Rahman, M.; Oparil, S.; Lewis, C.E.; et al. A randomized trial of intensive versus standard blood-pressure control. *N. Engl. J. Med.* **2015**, *373*, 2103–2116. [PubMed]
5. Zhang, W.; Zhang, S.; Deng, Y.; Wu, S.; Ren, J.; Sun, G.; Yang, J.; Jiang, Y.; Xu, X.; Wang, T.D.; et al. Trial of intensive blood-pressure control in older patients with hypertension. *N. Engl. J. Med.* **2021**, *385*, 1268–1279. [CrossRef]
6. Klahr, S.; Levey, A.S.; Beck, G.J.; Caggiula, A.W.; Hunsicker, L.; Kusek, J.W.; Striker, G. The effects of dietary protein restriction and blood-pressure control on the progression of chronic renal disease. Modification of diet in renal disease study group. *N. Engl. J. Med.* **1994**, *330*, 877–884. [CrossRef] [PubMed]
7. Ku, E.; Sarnak, M.J.; Toto, R.; McCulloch, C.E.; Lin, F.; Smogorzewski, M.; Hsu, C.Y. Effect of blood pressure control on long-term risk of end-stage renal disease and death among subgroups of patients with chronic kidney disease. *J. Am. Heart Assoc.* **2019**, *8*, e012749. [CrossRef] [PubMed]
8. Guerin, A.P.; Pannier, B.; Metivier, F.; Marchais, S.J.; London, G.M. Assessment and significance of arterial stiffness in patients with chronic kidney disease. *Curr. Opin. Nephro. L Hypertens.* **2008**, *17*, 635–641. [CrossRef]
9. Pannier, B.; Guerin, A.P.; Marchais, S.J.; Safar, M.E.; London, G.M. Stiffness of capacitive and conduit arteries: Prognostic significance for end-stage renal disease patients. *Hypertension* **2005**, *45*, 592–596. [CrossRef]
10. Van Bortel, L.M.; Laurent, S.; Boutouyrie, P.; Chowienczyk, P.; Cruickshank, J.K.; De Backer, T.; Filipovsky, J.; Huybrechts, S.; Mattace-Raso, F.U.; Protogerou, A.D.; et al. Expert consensus document on the measurement of aortic stiffness in daily practice using carotid-femoral pulse wave velocity. *J. Hypertens.* **2012**, *30*, 445–448. [CrossRef]
11. Spronck, B.; Terentes-Printzios, D.; Avolio, A.P.; Boutouyrie, P.; Guala, A.; Jerončić, A.; Laurent, S.; Barbosa, E.C.D.; Baulmann, J.; Chen, C.H.; et al. 2024 recommendations for validation of noninvasive arterial pulse wave velocity measurement devices. *Hypertension* **2024**, *81*, 183–192. [CrossRef]
12. Lin, W.C.; Wu, T.J.; Wang, C.H.; Hsieh, Y.J.; Hsu, B.G. Association between serum soluble urokinase-type plasminogen activator receptor level and arterial stiffness in chronic hemodialysis patients. *J. Pers. Med.* **2023**, *13*, 470. [CrossRef]
13. Huang, P.Y.; Hsu, B.G.; Lai, Y.H.; Wang, C.H.; Tsai, J.P. Serum trimethylamine N-oxide level is positively associated with aortic stiffness measured by carotid-femoral pulse wave velocity in patients undergoing maintenance hemodialysis. *Toxins* **2023**, *15*, 572. [CrossRef]
14. Coppack, S.W. Pro-inflammatory cytokines and adipose tissue. *Proc. Nutr. Soc.* **2001**, *60*, 349–356. [CrossRef] [PubMed]
15. Okamoto, Y.; Arita, Y.; Nishida, M.; Muraguchi, M.; Ouchi, N.; Takahashi, M.; Igura, T.; Inui, Y.; Kihara, S.; Nakamura, T.; et al. An adipocyte-derived plasma protein, adiponectin, adheres to injured vascular walls. *Horm. Metab. Res.* **2000**, *32*, 47–50. [CrossRef]
16. Ouchi, N.; Kihara, S.; Arita, Y.; Maeda, K.; Kuriyama, H.; Okamoto, Y.; Hotta, K.; Nishida, M.; Takahashi, M.; Nakamura, T.; et al. Novel modulator for endothelial adhesion molecules: Adipocyte-derived plasma protein adiponectin. *Circulation* **1999**, *100*, 2473–2476. [CrossRef]
17. Lassalle, P.; Molet, S.; Janin, A.; Heyden, J.V.; Tavernier, J.; Fiers, W.; Devos, R.; Tonnel, A.B. ESM-1 is a novel human endothelial cell-specific molecule expressed in lung and regulated by cytokines. *J. Biol. Chem.* **1996**, *271*, 20458–20464. [CrossRef]
18. Wellner, M.; Herse, F.; Janke, J.; Gorzelniak, K.; Engeli, S.; Bechart, D.; Lasalle, P.; Luft, F.C.; Sharma, A.M. Endothelial cell specific molecule-1—A newly identified protein in adipocytes. *Horm. Metab. Res.* **2003**, *35*, 217–221.

19. De Freitas Caires, N.; Gaudet, A.; Portier, L.; Tsicopoulos, A.; Mathieu, D.; Lassalle, P. Endocan, sepsis, pneumonia, and acute respiratory distress syndrome. *Crit. Care* **2018**, *22*, 280–289. [CrossRef] [PubMed]
20. Muhammad, I.F.; Borné, Y.; Östling, G.; Kennbäck, C.; Gottsäter, M.; Persson, M.; Nilsson, P.M.; Engström, G. Acute phase proteins as prospective risk markers for arterial stiffness: The Malmö Diet and Cancer cohort. *PLoS ONE* **2017**, *12*, e0181718. [CrossRef]
21. Zanoli, L.; Boutouyrie, P.; Fatuzzo, P.; Granata, A.; Lentini, P.; Oztürk, K.; Cappello, M.; Theocharidou, E.; Tuttolomondo, A.; Pinto, A.; et al. Inflammation and aortic Stiffness: An individual participant data meta-analysis in patients with inflammatory bowel disease. *J. Am. Heart Assoc.* **2017**, *6*, e007003–e007012. [CrossRef] [PubMed]
22. Khalaji, A.; Behnoush, A.H.; Mohtasham Kia, Y.; Alehossein, P.; Bahiraie, P. High circulating endocan in chronic kidney disease? A systematic review and meta-analysis. *PLoS ONE* **2023**, *18*, e0289710. [CrossRef] [PubMed]
23. Williams, B.; Mancia, G.; Spiering, W.; Agabiti Rosei, E.; Azizi, M.; Burnier, M.; Clement, D.L.; Coca, A.; de Simone, G.; Dominiczak, A.; et al. 2018 ESC/ESH Guidelines for the management of arterial hypertension. *Eur. Heart J.* **2018**, *39*, 3021–3104. [CrossRef] [PubMed]
24. Charra, B.; Chazot, C.; Jean, G.; Hurot, J.M.; Terrat, J.C.; Vanel, T.; Lorriaux, C.; Vovan, C. Role of sodium in dialysis. *Minerva Urol. Nefrol.* **2004**, *56*, 205–213. [PubMed]
25. Wanner, C.; Amann, K.; Shoji, T. The heart and vascular system in dialysis. *Lancet* **2016**, *388*, 276–284. [CrossRef] [PubMed]
26. Zoccali, C.; Moissl, U.; Chazot, C.; Mallamaci, F.; Tripepi, G.; Arkossy, O.; Wabel, P.; Stuard, S. Chronic fluid overload and mortality in ESRD. *J. Am. Soc. Nephrol.* **2017**, *28*, 2491–2497. [CrossRef] [PubMed]
27. Zanoli, L.; Lentini, P.; Briet, M.; Castellino, P.; House, A.A.; London, G.M.; Malatino, L.; McCullough, P.A.; Mikhailidis, D.P.; Boutouyrie, P. Arterial stiffness in the heart disease of CKD. *J. Am. Soc. Nephrol.* **2019**, *30*, 918–928. [CrossRef] [PubMed]
28. Hausberg, M.; Kosch, M.; Harmelink, P.; Barenbrock, M.; Hohage, H.; Kisters, K.; Dietl, K.H.; Rahn, K.H. Sympathetic nerve activity in end-stage renal disease. *Circulation* **2002**, *106*, 1974–1979. [CrossRef] [PubMed]
29. Kornerup, H.J.; Schmitz, O.; Danielsen, H.; Pedersen, E.B.; Giese, J. Significance of the renin-angiotensin system for blood pressure regulation in end-stage renal disease. *Contrib. Nephrol.* **1984**, *41*, 123–127.
30. Henrich, W.L.; Katz, F.H.; Molinoff, P.B.; Schrier, R.W. Competitive effects of hypokalemia and volume depletion on plasma renin activity, aldosterone and catecholamine concentrations in hemodialysis patients. *Kidney Int.* **1977**, *12*, 279–284. [CrossRef]
31. Calver, A.; Collier, J.; Leone, A.; Moncada, S.; Vallance, P. Effect of local intra-arterial asymmetric dimethylarginine (ADMA) on the forearm arteriolar bed of healthy volunteers. *J. Hum. Hypertens.* **1993**, *7*, 193–194. [PubMed]
32. Ramezanzadeh, E.; Fallah Arzpeyma, S.; Vakilpour, A.; Abedi, M.; Hassanipour, S. Endothelial function assessment by flow-mediated dilation of the brachial artery in acute kidney injury and chronic kidney disease. *Casp. J. Intern. Med.* **2023**, *14*, 668–675.
33. Morris, S.T.; McMurray, J.J.; Spiers, A.; Jardine, A.G. Impaired endothelial function in isolated human uremic resistance arteries. *Kidney Int.* **2001**, *60*, 1077–1082. [CrossRef] [PubMed]
34. Vaziri, N.D.; Ni, Z.; Oveisi, F.; Liang, K.; Pandian, R. Enhanced nitric oxide inactivation and protein nitration by reactive oxygen species in renal insufficiency. *Hypertension* **2002**, *39*, 135–141. [CrossRef] [PubMed]
35. Sieve, I.; Munster-Kuhnel, A.K.; Hilfiker-Kleiner, D. Regulation and function of endothelial glycocalyx layer in vascular diseases. *Vascul. Pharmacol.* **2018**, *100*, 26–33. [CrossRef] [PubMed]
36. Bar, A.; Targosz-Korecka, M.; Suraj, J.; Proniewski, B.; Jasztal, A.; Marczyk, B.; Sternak, M.; Przybyło, M.; Kurpińska, A.; Walczak, M.; et al. Degradation of glycocalyx and multiple manifestations of endothelial dysfunction coincide in the early phase of endothelial dysfunction before atherosclerotic plaque development in apolipoprotein E/low-density lipoprotein receptor-deficient mice. *J. Am. Heart Assoc.* **2019**, *8*, e011171. [CrossRef] [PubMed]
37. Sarrazin, S.; Adam, E.; Lyon, M.; Depontieu, F.; Motte, V.; Landolfi, C.; Lortat-Jacob, H.; Bechard, D.; Lassalle, P.; Delehedde, M. Endocan or endothelial cell specific molecule-1 (ESM-1): A potential novel endothelial cell marker and a new target for cancer therapy. *Biochim. Biophys. Acta* **2006**, *1765*, 25–37. [CrossRef]
38. Oka, S.; Obata, Y.; Sato, S.; Torigoe, K.; Sawa, M.; Abe, S.; Muta, K.; Ota, Y.; Kitamura, M.; Kawasaki, S.; et al. Serum endocan as a predictive marker for decreased urine volume in peritoneal dialysis patients. *Med. Sci. Monit.* **2017**, *23*, 1464–1470. [CrossRef]
39. Samouilidou, E.; Bountou, E.; Papandroulaki, F.; Papamanolis, M.; Papakostas, D.; Grapsa, E. Serum endocan levels are associated with paraoxonase 1 concentration in patients with chronic kidney disease. *Ther. Apher. Dial.* **2018**, *22*, 325–331. [CrossRef]
40. Bao, Y.; Wang, Y.A.; Xiao, H.; Wang, Y.; Wu, Y.; Yan, Y.; Zhu, Z.; Ni, M.; Pi, C.X.; Liu, M.Y.; et al. Serum endocan and circadian heart rate variability in non-dialysis stage 5 chronic kidney disease patients. *Int. Urol. Nephrol.* **2018**, *50*, 2061–2066. [CrossRef]
41. Poon, P.Y.; Ng, J.K.; Fung, W.W.; Chow, K.M.; Kwan, B.C.; Li, P.K.; Szeto, C.C. Relationship between Plasma Endocan Level and Clinical Outcome of Chinese Peritoneal Dialysis Patients. *Kidney Blood Press. Res.* **2019**, *44*, 1259–1270. [CrossRef] [PubMed]
42. Lin, J.H.; Hsu, B.G.; Wang, C.H.; Tsai, J.P. Endocan as a Potential Marker for Predicting All-Cause Mortality in Hemodialysis Patients. *J. Clin. Med.* **2023**, *12*, 7427. [CrossRef] [PubMed]
43. Kim, J.S.; Ko, G.J.; Kim, Y.G.; Lee, S.Y.; Lee, D.Y.; Jeong, K.H.; Lee, S.H. Plasma Endocan as a Predictor of Cardiovascular Event in Patients with End-Stage Renal Disease on Hemodialysis. *J. Clin. Med.* **2020**, *9*, 4086. [CrossRef] [PubMed]

44. Hureau, M.; Poissy, J.; Mathieu, D.; Dubucquoi, S.; Gaudet, A. Effects of intermittent hemodialysis on plasmatic levels of endocan. *Crit. Care.* **2021**, *25*, 412. [CrossRef] [PubMed]
45. Balta, S.; Balta, I.; Mikhailidis, D.P. Endocan: A new marker of endothelial function. *Curr. Opin. Cardiol.* **2021**, *36*, 462–468. [CrossRef]
46. Tian, X.; Zuo, Y.; Chen, S.; Zhang, Y.; Zhang, X.; Xu, Q.; Wu, S.; Wang, A. Hypertension, Arterial Stiffness, and Diabetes: A Prospective Cohort Study. *Hypertension* **2022**, *79*, 1487–1496. [CrossRef]

medicina

MDPI

Article

Coronary Artery Disease in Patients on Dialysis: Impact of Traditional Risk Factors

Dario Nakić [1,2], Petra Grbić Pavlović [1], Marina Vojković [1], Mira Stipćević [3], Jogen Patrk [3], Marin Bištirlić [3], Zoran Bakotić [3], Jelena Vučak Lončar [2,4] and Ivana Gusar [2,*]

[1] Department of Nephrology, General Hospital Zadar, Bože Peričića 5, 23000 Zadar, Croatia; dnakic@unizd.hr (D.N.); petricagrbic@hotmail.com (P.G.P.); marina.vojkovic03@gmail.com (M.V.)
[2] Department of Health Studies, University of Zadar, Splitska 1, 23000 Zadar, Croatia; jvucaklon@unizd.hr
[3] Department of Cardiology, General Hospital Zadar, Bože Peričića 5, 23000 Zadar, Croatia; mira.stipcevic@gmail.com (M.S.); jogen.patrk@bolnica-zadar.hr (J.P.); marin.bistirlic@gmail.com (M.B.); zbakotic@gmail.com (Z.B.)
[4] Department of Endocrinology, General Hospital Zadar, Bože Peričića 5, 23000 Zadar, Croatia
* Correspondence: igusar@unizd.hr; Tel.: +385-91-315-6785

Abstract: *Background and Objectives*: End-stage kidney disease (ESKD) is a major risk factor for cardiovascular morbidity and mortality. This study aims to evaluate the contribution of traditional risk factors to the development of coronary artery disease (CAD) in patients on dialysis. *Materials and Methods*: In this study, 54 patients on dialysis with angina symptoms or a positive exercise stress test underwent coronary angiography. Lesions with obstruction >70% lumen diameter of the coronary artery were considered significant. Traditional risk factors included hypertension, diabetes, smoking, dyslipidemia, age, gender, and time spent on dialysis. *Results*: Out of 54 participants, 41 (75.92%) were men and 13 (24.07%) women. CAD was present in 34 (62.96%) patients, and 20 (37.03%) patients were without CAD. The average age of the participants was 66.51 years. In the group with CAD, the average age was 69.52 years with an average time spent on dialysis of 2.73 years. In the group without CAD, the average age was 61.40 years with a time spent on dialysis of 2.35 years. Hypertension was present in 92.59% of all participants and 97.05% of those with CAD. Diabetes was present in 41.17 patients with CAD and 40% of those without CAD. Dyslipidemia was present in 76.47 participants with CAD and in 40% of those without CAD. Smoking was noticed in 35.29% of the participants with CAD and 57.14% of those without CAD. Besides hypertension, significant predictors for the development of CAD in patients on dialysis were dyslipidemia (OR 3.698, Cl 1.005–13.608, $p = 0.049$) and age (OR 1.056, Cl 1.004–1.110, $p = 0.033$). *Conclusions*: Among the traditional risk factors, hypertension, dyslipidemia, and age are the predictors for the development of CAD in patients on dialysis. Further large randomized clinical studies are needed to clarify the role of traditional risk factors for CAD in patients with ESKD.

Keywords: coronary artery disease; end-stage kidney disease; risk factors

1. Introduction

Cardiovascular disease (CVD) is the leading cause of morbidity and mortality among patients with end-stage kidney disease (ESKD) treated with the different modalities of dialysis. One of the most important manifestations of CVD in chronic kidney disease (CKD) is coronary artery disease (CAD). The prevalence of CAD and the number of significant coronary stenoses increases with the decrease in kidney function [1]. CVD results from traditional risk factors like hypertension, diabetes, dyslipidemia, smoking, and age, but also from non-traditional risk factors like arteriosclerosis, vascular calcifications, endothelial dysfunction, and low-grade inflammation [2,3]. Besides CAD, this process leads to left ventricular hypertrophy (LVH), diffuse fibrosis, left ventricular dilatation, and heart failure [4]. Cardiovascular mortality among patients on dialysis is 10–20 times higher compared to that of the general population of the same age and it is responsible for 50% of deaths among patients with ESKD [5]. According to the results from the US Kidney Data System, the prevalence of CAD in the CKD population is 39% versus 16% in the non-CKD population. The situation among patients undergoing hemodialysis is even worse, with the prevalence of CAD at 42% and that of CVD at 70% [6].

ESKD modifies the clinical presentation of the traditional symptoms of CAD. Acute myocardial infarction (AMI) with chest pain was presented in 44% of patients on dialysis compared with 68% of no-dialysis patients [7]. The recognition of CAD is more difficult with the persistence of anemia and fatigue common among patients on dialysis. Low functional capacity and achieving the threshold for angina pain also limit recognition of symptoms of angina pain in these patients [8]. Electrocardiogram (ECG) changes in angina pain are less common among patients on dialysis. A lower proportion of patients on dialysis presented with ST-segment changes than non-dialyzed patients. ECG changes are often present in patients with ESKD in the form of left ventricular hypertrophy (LVH), ST-segment, and T-wave abnormalities [9]. Serum biomarkers like cardiac troponin (high-sensitivity troponin-I and troponin-T) have limited sensitivity because they are often persistently elevated in patients with ESKD due to LVH, diastolic dysfunction, and volume overload in the absence of acute coronary syndrome [10].

Coronary angiography (CA) is considered the gold standard for diagnosing coronary stenosis in CAD. Coronary computed tomography angiography (CCTA) and coronary artery calcium score (CACS) might be used with caution in patients with ESKD, but the evidence comparing the accuracy of CCTA with CA in this population is limited. Low specificity could be explained by the high calcium burden in coronary arteries without significant stenosis [11,12]. Considering the limited number of studies on the development of coronary disease in dialysis patients and the presence of well-known risk factors, this study aimed to assess the presence and impact of traditional risk factors of coronary artery disease in dialysis patients. Traditional risk factors for CAD (hypertension, diabetes, dyslipidemia, smoking, and age) as well as time spent on dialysis were analyzed.

2. Materials and Methods

2.1. Study Design and Participants

This retrospective observational study was conducted for the period from 2019 to 2023. The patients included in this study were 54 adult patients over 18 years of age receiving dialysis: 51 on hemodialysis and 3 on peritoneal dialysis, all undergoing CA at a single center.

2.2. Data Collection

The age and gender of patients, as well as conventional cardiovascular risk factors (hypertension, diabetes, dyslipidemia, smoking, and history of peripheral vascular disease) and duration of dialysis, were collected from the patients' medical records.

2.3. Procedures

Inclusion indications for coronary angiography (CA) included angina symptoms or a positive exercise stress test (ergometry) in patients undergoing screening for kidney transplantation. Patients who did not have angina symptoms or had a negative exercise stress test (ergometry) were excluded from the study. Significant coronary artery lesions were considered significant if the stenosis was more than 70% of the luminal diameter.

CA was performed via the radial artery; only in cases where access via the radial artery was not possible was the femoral artery used. Lesions were coded according to the degree of obstruction, from normal to non-obstructive (<70% stenosis) and obstructive disease (>70% stenosis).

2.4. Statistical Analysis

Descriptive statistics for categorical variables are presented as proportions and percentages, while numerical data are presented with the mean and standard deviation. The ANOVA test was used to examine differences in the incidence of coronary artery disease concerning years of dialysis. Logistic regression was performed to identify predictors of coronary artery disease in dialysis patients. A significance level of $\alpha = 0.05$ was used as a criterion for the statistical significance of the results obtained. The data were analyzed using STATISTICA software version 14.0.0.15 (TIBCO Software Inc., Palo Alto, CA, USA, 2018).

3. Results

Of the 54 participants in the study, 41 (75.92%) were men and 13 (24.07%) were women. The most common underlying condition for ESKD was hypertensive/ischemic nephropathy (33%), diabetic nephropathy (28%), glomerulonephritis (22%), polycystic kidney disease (4%), and other conditions (13%). The average age of the participants was 66.51 years (SD = 13.12) (Table 1).

Table 1. Age of participants and duration of dialysis ($n = 54$).

Variable	Overall ($n = 54$)				Coronary Artery Disease ($n = 34$)				No Coronary Artery Disease ($n = 20$)				p
	Mean	**Min**	**Max**	**SD**	**Mean**	**Min**	**Max**	**SD**	**Mean**	**Min**	**Max**	**SD**	
Age *	66.51	29	90	13.12	69.52	38	90	10.93	61.40	29	89	15.13	0.026
Dialysis length *	2.59	1	11	2.12	2.73	1	11	2.15	2.35	1	7	2.10	0.526

Min—Minimum; Max—Maximum; * presented in years.

Participants who were diagnosed with coronary artery disease were older than participants who were not diagnosed with coronary artery disease ($p = 0.026$). The difference between participants regarding the duration of dialysis was not recorded ($p = 0.526$) (Table 1).

Most of the participants had a diagnosis of hypertension ($n = 50$; 92.59%), followed by dyslipidemia ($n = 36$; 66.66%). A total of 18 (33.33%) participants consumed tobacco products. More than half of the participants (32.96%) were found to have coronary artery disease on diagnostic coronary angiography (Figure 1).

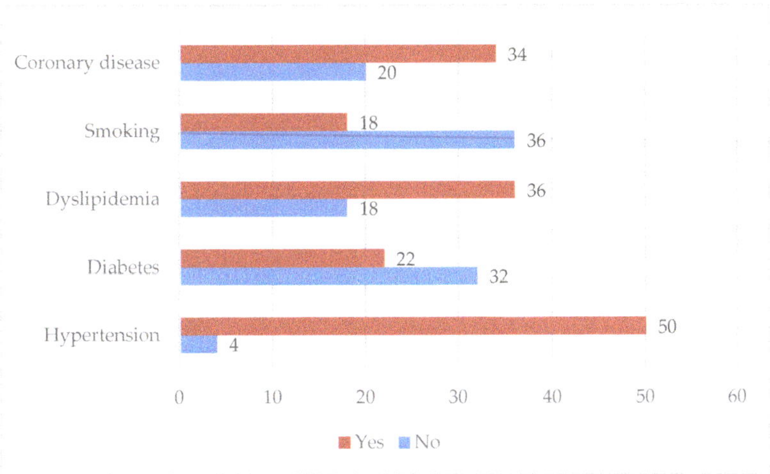

Figure 1. Characteristics of the participants concerning the presence of risk factors ($n = 54$).

The presence of hypertension was recorded in almost all participants diagnosed with coronary artery disease (n = 33), while a total of 26 patients with coronary artery disease were found to have dyslipidemia. The majority of participants diagnosed with coronary artery disease were men (n = 26) and most participants (n = 22) did not consume tobacco products (Table 2).

Table 2. Distribution and characteristics of participants with regard to the presence of coronary artery disease (n = 54).

Variable	**Coronary Artery Disease (n = 54)**				**Total**	
	Yes (n = 34)		**No (n = 20)**			
	Number	Percentage	Number	Percentage	Number	Percentage
Man	26	76.47	15	75.00	41	75.92
Woman	8	23.52	5	25.00	13	24.07
Hypertension	33	97.05	1	5.00	34	62.96
Diabetes	14	41.17	8	40.00	22	40.74
Dyslipidemia	26	76.47	8	40.00	34	62.96
Smoking	12	35.29	22	57.14	34	62.96

The results of the ANOVA test did not record a statistically significant difference (p = 0.120) in the incidence of coronary disease among the participants regarding the duration of dialysis. Therefore, the duration of dialysis, as well as the presence of hypertension due to its presence in almost all subjects with coronary artery disease, was excluded from further analysis.

After applying logistic regression analysis, age (OR 1.056, 95% Cl 1.004–1.110, p = 0.033) and dyslipidemia (OR 3.698, 95% Cl 1.005–13.608, p = 0.049) were recorded as statistically significant predictors of coronary artery disease in the participants of this study. With an increase of one year of life, the chance of coronary disease increased 1.05 times. Furthermore, participants diagnosed with dyslipidemia had a 3.69 times higher risk of developing coronary artery disease (Table 3).

Table 3. Logistic regression analysis for predictors of coronary artery disease in dialysis patients (n = 54).

Variable	**B**	**S.E.**	**Wald**	**df**	**p ***	**OR**	**95% CL**	
							Lower	**Upper**
Age	0.055	0.026	4.547	1	0.033	1.056	1.004	1.110
Diabetes	−0.003	0.654	0.000	1	0.997	0.997	0.277	3.595
Dyslipidemia	1.308	0.665	3.872	1	0.049	3.698	1.005	13.608
Smoking	0.526	0.680	0.598	1	0.439	1.692	0.447	6.409
Constant	−4.084	1.914	4.553	1	0.033	0.017		

* Logistic regression analysis.

4. Discussion

Patients with ESRD who require dialysis have a significantly increased risk of morbidity and mortality from CVD. CAD is the major clinical manifestation of a worse prognosis for these patients. It is more likely to develop acute myocardial infarction (AMI) than stable angina as an initial clinical manifestation of CAD. AMI is more likely to be a non-ST-segment elevation myocardial infarction (nSTEMI) than an ST-segment elevation myocardial infarction (STEMI) [13,14]. Relatively common in dialysis patients is a sudden death perhaps because of changes in electrolytes, volume, and drug concentration which may trigger arrhythmias in patients with LVH and heart failure, which are common in these patients [4].

Hypertension is the most common CVD risk factor in patients with ESKD. In our study group, it was present in 92% of all participants and in 97% of those with CAD, which confirms hypertension as the most important risk factor for CAD not only in patients with ESKD. Similar results were found in the study by Vasuveda et al. in patients with stable CAD and ESKD who underwent coronary artery bypass grafting (CABG) with a hypertension prevalence of 97% [15]. In a study on predictors of CAD progression in high-risk patients with recurrent symptoms, Fatah et al. reported a 71% prevalence of hypertension [16].

In addition, this study found that dyslipidemia is an important risk factor for the development of CAD in ESKD patients, increasing the risk by 3.69 times. The treatment of dyslipidemia in patients with ESKD is controversial. The benefit of statin-based treatment in reducing serious vascular events is lower with the decline in the glomerular filtration rate, with no clear evidence for dialysis patients [17].

Also, age was found to be a risk factor for the development of CAD in patients on dialysis with a chance of developing CAD of 1.05 per year. This was not noticed for the years spent on dialysis. Chen et al. found, in a study of Asian dialysis patients, that higher all-cause mortality was associated with a dialysis time greater than 3 years in patients undergoing CABG [18]. In this study, both groups, with and without CAD, spent less than 3 years on dialysis; those with CAD spent 2.73 years and those without CAD spent 2.35 years on dialysis, which may suggest that a much longer duration of dialysis may be associated with a higher risk of developing CAD.

Diabetes mellitus (DM) and chronic kidney disease (CKD) are among the strongest risk factors for cardiovascular disease (CVD) [19]. This includes every aspect of CVD, including atherosclerotic CVD (ASCVD), heart failure (HF), valvular heart disease, peripheral arterial disease (PAD), stroke, and arrhythmias [20]. In addition, the overall mortality associated with CVD in these conditions remains high. The coexistence of these conditions has additive and sometimes multiplicative effects on these outcomes [21]. Based on the results of this study, 41.17% of patients with CAD were diabetic patients, but 40% without CAD had diabetes as an additional risk factor, so we found no association between diabetes and the risk of CAD in patients on dialysis.

According to the literature, smoking increases all causes of death in dialysis patients and leads to a 10-year reduction in life expectancy. It also leads to a 36% higher risk of cardiovascular events [22,23]. It is important to emphasize that several studies have found that smoking increases the incidence of peripheral vascular events and heart failure. However, an increased incidence of cerebrovascular or coronary vascular events was not found [24]. Furthermore, smoking accelerates atherosclerotic disease, impairs endothelial function, increases blood pressure, and increases sympathetic outflow [23]. Smoking before dialysis causes acute elevations in blood pressure, leading to more antihypertensive medications being prescribed which interfere with adequate fluid withdrawal due to intradialytic hypotension [23]. In this study, 35% of patients were active smokers, which is a significantly higher percentage than the results found in the literature (15%) [22], but is very similar to the results of 31% of smokers from reports of previous Croatian epidemiological studies in the general population [25]. An association between smoking and the progression of coronary artery disease in smokers among the dialysis population was not found in this study.

There are different treatment options for CAD in advanced CKD: conservative and interventional strategies such as percutaneous coronary intervention (PCI) and coronary artery bypass grafting (CABG) [26]. Reports from the ISCHEMIA-CKD trial provided no evidence that the initial invasive strategy reduced the risk of death or non-fatal myocardial infarction in these patients compared with the initial conservative strategy [27]. For the invasive approach, there is still no clear evidence of the benefits of CABG or PCI. In the SYNTAX trial [28], there is an advantage of CABG, EXCEL showed no significant difference between PCI and CABG [29], and in a national study from Taiwan, PCI with a drug-eluting stent was associated with better survival in dialysis patients [30].

Among patients on dialysis, there is a high prevalence of asymptomatic patients, estimated to be between 42 and 54% according to some reports [31]. The KDIGO guidelines for cardiovascular disease in dialysis patients recommend annual CAD evaluation in patients with diabetes on the waiting list for transplantation as a non-invasive screening [32]. Currently, routine invasive screening for CAD is not part of clinical practice for these patients. However, in the future, it may be necessary to consider implementing this option to prevent CAD and promptly improve dialysis patients' treatment. Although this study provides valuable results and information that may potentially contribute to deciding on the introduction of additional preventive diagnostic procedures for dialysis patients, the fact that this is a relatively small sample of patients from a single healthcare institution that cares for the population of a relatively limited geographical area should also be taken into account. Furthermore, we did not collect other parameters of prognostic value in this study, such as laboratory measurements and pharmacotherapy, which may also have a significant impact on patient outcomes.

5. Conclusions

Hypertension, dyslipidemia, and age were significant predictors for the development of CAD in patients on dialysis, and better control of hypertension and dyslipidemia is necessary to prevent the occurrence of CAD in these patients. Further large randomized clinical trials are needed to clarify the role of traditional risk factors for CAD in patients with ESKD.

Author Contributions: Conceptualization, D.N., P.G.P., M.V., M.S., J.P., M.B., Z.B., J.V.L. and I.G.; methodology, D.N., P.G.P., M.V., M.S., J.P., M.B., Z.B. and I.G.; software, D.N. and I.G.; validation, D.N., P.G.P., M.V., M.S. and J.P.; formal analysis, D.N. and I.G.; investigation, D.N., P.G.P., M.V., M.S., J.P., M.B., Z.B. and J.V.L.; resources, D.N., M.S., J.P., M.B. and Z.B.; data curation, D.N., P.G.P., M.V., M.S., J.P., M.B., Z.B. and J.V.L.; writing—original draft preparation, D.N., P.G.P., M.V., M.S., J.P., M.B., Z.B., J.V.L. and I.G.; writing—review and editing, D.N., P.G.P., M.V., M.S., J.P., M.B., Z.B., J.V.L. and I.G.; visualization, D.N. and I.G.; supervision, J.P.; project administration, D.N. All authors have read and agreed to the published version of the manuscript.

Funding: This research received no external funding.

Institutional Review Board Statement: This study was conducted in accordance with the Declaration of Helsinki and the recommendations of the Institutional Ethics Committee of General Hospital Zadar (Approval Code: 01-5661/12-9/24; Approval Date: 3 June 2024).

Informed Consent Statement: All data are available from the corresponding author upon reasonable request.

Data Availability Statement: The authors will make available the data supporting this article's conclusions on request.

Acknowledgments: We thank all of the participants who participated in this study.

Conflicts of Interest: The authors declare no conflicts of interest.

References

1. Fujii, H.; Kono, K.; Nishi, S. Characteristics of coronary artery disease in chronic kidney disease. *Clin. Exp. Nephrol.* **2019**, *23*, 725–732. [CrossRef]
2. Gansevoort, R.T.; Correa-Rotter, R.; Hemmelgarn, B.R.; Jafar, T.H.; Heerspink, H.J.; Mann, J.F.; Matsushita, K.; Wen, C.P. Chronic kidney disease and cardiovascular risk: Epidemiology, mechanisms, and prevention. *Lancet* **2013**, *382*, 339–352. [CrossRef] [PubMed]
3. Burton, J.O.; Jefferies, H.J.; Selby, N.M.; McIntyre, C.W. Hemodialysis-induced cardiac injury: Determinants and associated outcomes. *Clin. J. Am. Soc. Nephrol.* **2009**, *4*, 914–920. [CrossRef] [PubMed]
4. Wanner, C.; Amann, K.; Shoji, T. The heart and vascular system in dialysis. *Lancet* **2016**, *388*, 276–284. [CrossRef] [PubMed]
5. Poli, F.E.; Gulsin, G.S.; McCann, G.P.; Burton, J.O.; Graham-Brown, M.P. The assessment of coronary artery disease on patients with end-stage renal disease. *Clin. Kidney J.* **2019**, *12*, 721–734. [CrossRef] [PubMed]

6. Li, X.; Xiao, F.; Zhang, S. Coronary revascularisation in patients with chronic kidney disease and end-stage renal disease: A meta-analysis. *Int. J. Clin. Pract.* **2021**, *75*, e14506. [CrossRef] [PubMed]
7. Herzog, C.A.; Littrell, K.; Arko, C.; Frederick, P.D.; Blaney, M. Clinical characteristics of dialysis patients with acute myocardial infarction in the United States: A collaborative project of the United States Renal Data System and the National Registry of Myocardial Infarction. *Circulation* **2007**, *116*, 1465–1472. [CrossRef] [PubMed]
8. Sarnak, M.J.; Amann, K.; Bangalore, S.; Cavalcante, J.L.; Charytan, D.M.; Craig, J.C.; Gill, J.S.; Hlatky, M.A.; Jardine, A.G.; Landmesser, U.; et al. Conference Participants. Chronic kidney disease and coronary artery disease. *J. Am. Coll. Cardiol.* **2019**, *74*, 1823–1838. [CrossRef] [PubMed]
9. Abe, S.; Yoshizawa, M.; Nakanishi, N.; Yazawa, T.; Yokota, K.; Honda, M.; Sloman, G. Electrocardiographic abnormalities in patients receiving hemodialysis. *Am. Heart J.* **1996**, *131*, 1137–1144. [CrossRef]
10. Mahajan, V.S.; Jarolim, P. How to interpret elevated cardiac troponin levels. *Circulation* **2011**, *124*, 2350–2354. [CrossRef]
11. Mao, J.; Karthikeyan, V.; Poopat, C.; Song, T.; Pantelic, M.; Chattahi, J.; Cavalcante, J.L.; Ananthasubramaniam, K. Coronary computed tomography angiography in dialysis patients undergoing pre-renal transplantation cardiac risk stratification. *Cardiol. J.* **2010**, *17*, 349–361.
12. Jug, B.; Kadakia, J.; Gupta, M.; Papazian, J.; Derakhshani, A.; Koplik, S.; Karlsberg, R.P.; Budoff, M.J. Coronary calcifications and plaque characteristics in patients with end-stage renal disease: A computed tomography study. *Coron. Artery Dis.* **2013**, *24*, 501–508. [CrossRef]
13. Go, A.S.; Bansal, N.; Chandra, M.; Lathon, P.V.; Fortmann, S.P.; Iribarren, C.; Hsu, C.Y.; Hlatky, M.A.; ADVANCE Study Investigators. Chronic kidney disease and risk for presenting with acute myocardial infarction versus stable exertional angina in adults with coronary heart disease. *J. Am. Coll. Cardiol.* **2011**, *58*, 1600–1607. [CrossRef]
14. Shroff, G.R.; Li, S.; Herzog, C.A. Trends in discharge claims for acute myocardial infarction among patients on dialysis. *J. Am. Soc. Nephrol.* **2017**, *28*, 1379–1383. [CrossRef]
15. Vasudeva, R.; Mehta, H.; Chan, W.C.; Majmundar, M.; Yarlagadda, S.G.; Downey, P.; Daon, E.; Muehlebach, G.; Danter, M.; Zorn, G.; et al. Trends and outcomes for coronary artery bypass grafting in end-stage kidney disease and stable coronary artery disease. *Am. J. Cardiol.* **2024**, *1*, 37–43. [CrossRef]
16. Farah, I.; Ahmed, A.M.; Odeh, R.; Alameen, E.; Al-Khateeb, M.; Fadel, E.; Rabai, R.; Ali, D.; Bdeir, B.; Al-Mallah, M.H. Predictors of coronary artery disease progression among high-risk patients with recurrent symptoms. *Heart Views* **2018**, *19*, 45–48. [CrossRef]
17. Fellström, B.; Holdaas, H.; Jardine, A.G.; Rose, H.; Schmieder, R.; Wilpshaar, W.; Zannad, F.; AURORA Study Group. Effect of rosuvastatin on outcomes in chronic haemodialysis patients: Baseline dana from the AURORA study. *Kidney Blood Pres. Res.* **2007**, *30*, 314–322. [CrossRef]
18. Chen, S.W.; Chang, C.H.; Lin, Y.S.; Wu, V.C.; Chen, D.Y.; Tsai, F.C.; Hung, M.J.; Chu, P.H.; Lin, P.J.; Chen, T.H. Effect of dialysis dependence and duration on post-coronary artery bypass grafting outcomes in patients with chronic kidney disease: A nationwide cohort study in Asia. *Int. J. Cardiol.* **2016**, *223*, 65–71. [CrossRef]
19. Zhao, Y.; Malik, S.; Budoff, M.J.; Correa, A.; Ashley, K.E.; Selvin, E.; Watson, K.E.; Wong, N.D. Identification and predictors for cardiovascular disease risk equivalents among adults with diabetes mellitus. *Diabetes Care* **2021**, *44*, 2411–2418. [CrossRef] [PubMed]
20. Pop-Busui, R.; Januzzi, J.L.; Bruemmer, D.; Butalia, S.; Green, J.B.; Horton, W.B.; Knight, C.; Levi, M.; Rasouli, N.; Richardson, C.R. Heart failure: An underappreciated complication of diabetes. A consensus report of the American Diabetes Association. *Diabetes Care* **2022**, *45*, 1670–1690. [CrossRef] [PubMed]
21. Papademetriou, V.; Lovato, L.; Doumas, M.; Nylen, E.; Mottl, A.; Cohen, R.M.; Applegate, W.B.; Puntakee, Z.; Yale, J.F.; Cushman, W.C. Chronic kidney disease and intensive glycemic control increase cardiovascular risk in patients with type 2 diabetes. *Kidney Int.* **2015**, *87*, 649–659. [CrossRef]
22. Li, N.C.; Thadhani, R.I.; Reviriego-Mendoza, M.; Larkin, J.W.; Maddux, F.W.; Ofsthun, N.J. Association of smoking status with mortality and hospitalization in hemodialysis patients. *Am. J. Kidney Dis.* **2018**, *72*, 673–681. [CrossRef]
23. Tapolyai, M.; Forró, M.; Lengvárszky, Z.; Fülöp, T. Dialysis patient who smoke are more hypertensive, more fluid overloaded and take more antihypertensive medications than nonsmokers. *Ren. Fail.* **2020**, *42*, 413–418. [CrossRef]
24. Liebman, S.E.; Lamontagne, S.P.; Huang, L.S.; Messing, S.; Bushinsky, D.A. Smoking in Dialysis Patients: A Systematic Review and Meta-analysis of Mortality and Cardiovascular Morbidity. *Am. J. Kidney Dis.* **2011**, *58*, 257–265. [CrossRef]
25. Nakić, D.; Stipčević, M.; Morić Perić, M.; Bakotić, Z.; Lončar, J.V.; Bačkov, K.; Vojković, M.; Jakab, J.; Včev, A. Chronic medical conditions in Croatian war veterans compared to general popolation: 25 years after the war. *Acta Clin. Croat.* **2023**, *62*, 3–10. [CrossRef]
26. Losin, I.; Hagai, K.C.; Pereg, D. The treatment of coronary artery disease in patients with chronic kidney disease: Gaps, challenges, and solutions. *Kidney Dis.* **2023**, *10*, 12–22. [CrossRef]
27. Bangalore, S.; Maron, D.J.; O'Brien, S.M.; Fleg, J.L.; Kretov, E.I.; Briguori, C.; Kaul, U.; Reynolds, H.R.; Mazurek, T.; Sidhu, M.S.; et al. Management of coronary disease in patients with advanced kidney disease. *N. Engl. J. Med.* **2020**, *382*, 1608–1618. [CrossRef]
28. Milojevic, M.; Head, S.J.; Mack, M.J.; Mohr, F.W.; Morice, M.C.; Dawkins, K.D.; Holmes, D.R., Jr.; Serruys, P.W.; Kappetein, A.P. The impact of chronic kidney disease on outcomes following percutaneous coronary intervention versus coronary artery bypass grafting in patients with complex coronary artery disease: Five-year follow-up of the SYNTAX trial. *Eurointervention* **2018**, *14*, 102–111. [CrossRef]

29. Giustino, G.; Mehran, R.; Serruys, P.W.; Sabik, J.F.; Milojevic, M., 3rd; Simonton, C.A.; Puskas, J.D.; Kandzari, D.E.; Morice, M.C.; Taggart, D.P.; et al. Left main revascularization with PCI or CABG in patients with chronic kidney disease: EXCEL trial. *J. Am. Coll. Cardiol.* **2018**, *72*, 754–765. [CrossRef] [PubMed]
30. Pan, S.Y.; Yang, J.Y.; Teng, N.C.; Chen, Y.Y.; Wang, S.H.; Lee, C.L.; Chen, K.L.; Chiu, Y.L.; Hsu, S.P.; Peng, Y.S.; et al. Percutaneous coronary intervention with a drug-eluting stent versus coronary artery bypass grafting in patients receiving dialysis: A national study from Taiwan. *Kidney Med.* **2023**, *6*, 100768. [CrossRef] [PubMed]
31. De Vriese, A.S.; Vandecasteele, S.J.; Van den Bergh, B.; De Geeter, F.W. Should we screen for coronary artery disease in asymptomatic chronic dialysis patients? *Kidney Int.* **2012**, *81*, 143–151. [CrossRef] [PubMed]
32. Kidney Disease: Improving Global Outcomes (KDIGO) CKD Work Group. KDIGO 2024 Clinical Practice Guideline for the Evaluation and Management of Chronic Kidney Disease. *Kidney Int.* **2024**, *105*, S117–S314. [CrossRef] [PubMed]

medicina MDPI

Article

Echocardiographic Indices in Patients with End-Stage Renal Disease and Their Association with Hemodialysis-to-Hemodiafiltration Transfer: A Prospective Observational Study

Josipa Domjanović Matetić [1], Darija Baković Kramarić [2], Tea Domjanović Škopinić [2], Ivo Jeličić [1], Dijana Borić Škaro [1], Joško Božić [3,4] and Andrija Matetic [2,4,*]

[1] Department of Nephrology, University Hospital of Split, 21000 Split, Croatia; josipa.domjanovic@gmail.com (J.D.M.); ivo.jelicic@gmail.com (I.J.); zanaboric@gmail.com (D.B.Š.)
[2] Department of Cardiology, University Hospital of Split, 21000 Split, Croatia; darija.bakovic@mefst.hr (D.B.K.); tea.domjanovic@gmail.com (T.D.Š.)
[3] Department of Pathophysiology, University of Split School of Medicine, 21000 Split, Croatia; josko.bozic@mefst.hr
[4] University of Split School of Medicine, 21000 Split, Croatia
* Correspondence: andrija.matetic@gmail.com

Abstract: *Background and Objectives*: The assessment of cardiac function in patients with end-stage renal disease (ESRD) is vital due to their high cardiovascular risk. However, contemporary echocardiographic indices and their association with hemodialysis-to-hemodiafiltration transfer are underreported in this population. *Materials and Methods*: This prospective cohort study enrolled 36 ESRD patients undergoing hemodialysis-to-hemodiafiltration transfer, with baseline and 3-month post-transfer comprehensive echocardiographic assessments. The key parameters included the global work index, global constructed work, global wasted work (GWW), global work efficiency (GWE), and global longitudinal strain (GLS), with secondary measures from conventional echocardiography. The baseline measures were compared to general population reference values and changes pre- to post-transfer were analyzed using the Mann–Whitney U test. *Results*: Patients exhibited significant deviations from reference ranges in GWW (179.0 vs. 53.0–122.2 mmHg%), GWE (90.0 vs. 53.0–122.2%), and GLS (−16.0 vs. −24.0–(−16.0)%). Post-transfer left ventricular myocardial work and longitudinal strain remained unchanged ($p > 0.05$), except for increased GWW (179.0, IQR 148.0–217.0 to 233.5, IQR 159.0-315.0 mmHg%, $p = 0.037$) and improved mid-inferior peak systolic longitudinal strain ((−17.0, IQR −19.0–(−11.0) to −18.7, IQR −20.0–(−18.0)%, $p = 0.016$). The enrolled patients also showed higher left atrial diameters, left ventricular volumes, and mass, with impaired systolic function in both ventricles compared to reference values. *Conclusions*: This study highlights baseline impairments in contemporary echocardiographic measures (GWW, GWE, GLS) in ESRD patients versus reference values, but found no association between hemodialysis-to-hemodiafiltration transfer and most myocardial work and strain parameters.

Keywords: end-stage renal disease; hemodialysis; hemodiafiltration; contemporary echocardiography

1. Introduction

End-stage renal disease (ESRD) is a major global health burden with substantial cardiovascular complications and increased cardiovascular mortality [1,2]. These patients exhibit several negative cardiovascular risk factors, such as accelerated atherosclerosis due to chronic inflammation [2], enhanced vascular and valvular calcifications resulting from impaired mineral metabolism [2,3], and cardiac dysfunction driven by increased loading conditions [4]. Additionally, negative cardiovascular effects may be associated with dialysis that carries proinflammatory response, intradialytic hypotension [5], cardiac load oscillations, and impaired myocardial perfusion [5,6].

As a result, there is a growing trend toward timely stratification of cardiovascular function in ESRD patients, but also toward transitioning patients to newer dialytic modalities like hemodiafiltration, which may offer cardiovascular benefits [1,7,8]. Hemodiafiltration allows a more effective removal of harmful proinflammatory and proatherogenic substances, such as β2-microglobulin, cytokines, advanced glycation end products, and fibroblast growth factors [9,10]. Although the removal of these middle-weight molecules could mitigate negative cardiovascular effects, their impact on cardiovascular tests such as echocardiography is still unclear.

Echocardiography is an essential diagnostic method in patients with ESRD due to its non-invasiveness and availability. Contemporary echocardiographic analyses such as myocardial work and strain imaging enable the detection of subtle cardiac changes and may potentially allow for earlier therapeutic intervention in this vulnerable population. Importantly, previous studies have reported an association of advanced echocardiographic measures such as the left ventricular strain with mortality in pre-dialysis [11], stable hemodialysis [12], and overall ESRD patients [13], with worse function being associated with impaired prognosis. Their predictive performance was shown to be superior to standard echocardiographic measures like the left ventricular ejection fraction [14], further emphasizing their clinical importance and the need for further evaluation amongst patients with ESRD. However, contemporary echocardiographic data are generally underreported in ESRD patients, and there is an unmet need for their better understanding, particularly in the context of established reference ranges and different dialysis modalities.

Therefore, this study aimed to describe the contemporary echocardiographic measures in patients with ESRD and determine their association with the hemodialysis-to-hemodiafiltration transfer, using the comprehensive echocardiographic analyses. Importantly, this study has an important hypothesis-generating purpose to support further research and stimulate the development of novel diagnostic and therapeutic modalities in these settings.

2. Materials and Methods

2.1. Ethical and Reporting Considerations

This study was approved by the Ethics Committee of the University Hospital of Split, Croatia (Date of approval: 28 May 2021; No. 2181-147/01/06/M.S.-21-02). All participants completed an informed consent form. All the proceedings and clinical research were performed with the ethical standards of the Declaration of Helsinki and its amendments. The Strengthening the Reporting of Observational Studies in Epidemiology (STROBE) checklist for observational studies is reported in Supplementary STROBE Statement.

2.2. Study Design and Participants

This longitudinal prospective observational study enrolled a total of 36 consecutive adult patients (≥18 years) with ESRD who were scheduled for a planned therapeutic hemodialysis-to-hemodiafiltration transfer at the Department of Nephrology and Hemodialysis at the University Hospital of Split over the period from September 2021 to January 2023. The main eligibility criteria for the hemodialysis-to-hemodiafiltration transfer were defined solely on the institutional protocol, including the: regular management with conventional hemodialysis for at least 6 months (3 times a week); stable efficiency parameters (minimal single-pool Kt/V for urea of 1.2); and availability of adequate vascular access. The exclusion criteria were as follows: known or established valvular heart disease; active malignant disease; and poor echocardiographic acoustic window. For the purpose of this research study, the authors did not consider any other eligibility/exclusion criteria. The flow diagram of the study is shown in Supplementary Figure S1.

2.3. Data Sources

Detailed patient data were collected from the medical records, while other measurements were performed according to applicable medical standards. All anthropometric measurements were determined according to the recommendations of the World Health Organization, including the measurement of body height, body weight, and body mass index (BMI) [15]. Importantly, all medication regimens were stably maintained during the study period.

Routine laboratory analysis was conducted according to the standard protocols of the Department of Nephrology and Hemodialysis at the University Hospital of Split. Venous blood was sampled by a trained medical technician/nurse from the dialytic system (up to 22 mL of blood) at different time points, including the last hemodialysis session (before and after the hemodialysis session) and 3 months after the hemodialysis-to-hemodiafiltration transfer (before and after the hemodiafiltration session).

2.4. Conventional Hemodialysis

Conventional hemodialysis was performed using the universal machine in our centre (Fresenius 5008; Fresenius SE & Co., Hochtaunuskreis, Germany) with poly-sulfone membranes and blood flow of 300 mL/min. The dialyzers used for conventional hemodialysis were Fx60 (Fresenius SE & Co., Hochtaunuskreis, Germany), Fx80 (Fresenius SE & Co., Hochtaunuskreis, Germany), Leoceed-16N (Asahi Kasei Corp., Tokyo, Japan), and Nipro 150 (Nipro Medical Europe, Mechelen, Belgium).

2.5. Hemodiafiltration

The on-line hemodiafiltration in this study was performed using the hemodiafiltration machine (Fresenius 5008) with poly-sulfone membranes containing >23 L of convective volume; blood flow of 300 to 350 mL/min; and dialysate flow of 500–600 mL/min. The dialyzers used for hemodiafiltration were Fx60 and Fx80.

Both hemodialysis and hemodiafiltration treatment modalities were performed using the ultrapure dialysates as defined by bacterial counts <0.1/mL colony-forming units (CFU) and <0.025 units of endotoxin per mL.

2.6. Comprehensive Echocardiographic Assessment

The transthoracic echocardiographic examinations were performed by a single highly experienced cardiologist specialized in cardiac imaging, per standard echocardiographic protocols [16]. Echocardiographic imaging was conducted using the advanced ultrasound system (Vivid 9E; GE Healthcare, Chicago, IL, USA). Data were digitally stored and analyzed on the Echo PAC workstation (Echo PAC 202 PC; GE Healthcare, Chicago, IL, USA).

Echocardiography assessments were always performed on the non-dialysis days before the mid-week hemodialysis or hemodiafiltration. Measurements were collected at 2 time points: baseline measurement (before the hemodialysis-to-hemodiafiltration transfer), and control measurement (3 months after the hemodialysis-to-hemodiafiltration transfer).

The echocardiographic analysis included standard 2-dimensional echocardiographic projections (parasternal long and short axis-view; apical 4, 5 and 3-chamber view) and additional modified views if necessary. Obtained images were used to measure standard 2-dimensional dimensions (left atrium, left ventricle, interventricular septum, posterior wall of the left ventricle, aortic root and ascending aorta) and to calculate 2-dimensional ejection fraction using Simpson's biplane method. Left atrial volume and left ventricular mass were standardized according to body surface area (BSA). The 4-dimensional probe was used to obtain multi-slice images of the left ventricle and to derive 4-dimensional left ventricular volumes. Valves were analyzed morphologically and functionally using Doppler echocardiography. Using the pulse wave and tissue Doppler echocardiography, parameters of left ventricular diastolic function were evaluated—E and A wave velocity, E/A ratio, E wave deceleration time, and e and e' velocity. These measurements were combined with left atrial indexed volume and tricuspid velocity to determine the degree of diastolic dysfunction.

Using the apical projections, global longitudinal strain by speckle tracking echocardiography and myocardial work were determined to evaluate left ventricular function. Myocardial work is a pressure-dependent echocardiographic measure of left ventricular function that relies on the pressure–strain loop, thereby reducing its dependence on the afterload conditions [17]. It can be further divided into global work index (GWI), global constructive work (GCW), global wasted work (GWW), and global work efficiency (GWE). GWI represents total left ventricular work, GCW represents systolic shortening of cardiomyocyte and stretching during isovolumic relaxation, GWW represents systolic stretching of cardiomyocyte and shortening during isovolumic relaxation, and GWE is calculated from GCW divided with sum of GCW and GWW [18]. The protocol for myocardial work assessment included the utilization of Automated Functional Imaging (AFI) and its myocardial work module on Echo PAC 202 PC software. The echocardiographer entered the blood pressure values (systolic cuff pressure measurement) and valvular event times (time from mitral valve closure to mitral valve opening) to the predefined areas within the software. These data were utilized by the software to compute the global myocardial work (average of all segmental values) but also to determine the segmental work as strain–pressure loops.

Left ventricular strain imaging evaluates the global and segmental myocardial deformation, which is related to cardiac contractility and fibrosis [19]. There are 3 types of myocardial strain, including the longitudinal, radial, and circumferential strain. All strain types are dependent on cardiomyocyte shortening and represent left ventricular systolic function [5]. The left ventricular longitudinal strain was performed using the AFI on Echo PAC 202 PC software. After obtaining three standard apical views (apical long-axis, four and two chamber), the apical long-axis view was used to define end-systole by closure of the aortic valve. Subsequently, three index points of mitral annulus and left ventricular apex were defined in each of the views at end-systole. Endocardium borders, i.e., speckles within the endocardium, are automatically traced and tracked during the entire cardiac cycle. The software then automatically defines changes in length of the tracked speckle, where lengthening (during diastole) is expressed as positive value and shortening (during systole) is expressed as negative value. The difference between the end-diastolic and end-systolic value is divided with the original reference length giving the value of strain expressed in percentage. This is performed for each region of the myocardium and the software at the end provides a bullseye of the left ventricle giving us values of LS for each of the segments and also the average value, known as global longitudinal strain. In case the automatic endocardial border tracking is not correct, the echocardiographer can readjust the region of interest and recalculate the values.

The right ventricle was evaluated using the standard 2-dimensional and 4-dimensional probe standard (parasternal long-axis view; apical 4-chamber view) and modified apical projections for the right ventricle. Furthermore, the 4D probe was used to obtain multi-slice images of the right ventricle that were then used for volumetric measurements.

2.7. Outcomes

The main outcome of this study was the comparison of echocardiographic measurements about hemodialysis-to-hemodiafiltration transfer (baseline vs. 3-month follow-up values). The secondary outcome included the comparison of baseline echocardiographic measurements to reference values from the general population (median values vs. reference values). Other outcomes were laboratory parameters and the efficacy of dialysis regarding the hemodialysis-to-hemodiafiltration transfer (baseline vs. 3-month follow-up values).

2.8. Statistical Analysis

Statistical data analysis was carried out using a Statistical Package for the Social Sciences (SPSS) software (IBM Corp, NY, USA; version 20). Continuous data were presented as median (interquartile range [IQR]), while categorical variables were expressed as numbers (percentages). This analysis used non-parametric tests, such as the Mann–Whitney test, as they do not assume a specific distribution of the data, making it more robust and reliable in analyses with limited sample sizes. The baseline echocardiographic measurements were compared to the general population by evaluating the deviation of the median from the established reference ranges for each echocardiographic parameter, as defined by the Normal Reference Ranges for Echocardiography (NORRE) of the European Association of Cardiovascular Imaging (EACVI) and other relevant studies [16,20–25]. Additional data analysis was performed to determine the 95% confidence intervals (95%CI) and compare them with the established reference ranges for the main left ventricular myocardial work and longitudinal strain parameters. To test the within-subjects differences in echocardiographic measurements over the follow-up, we used the Mann–Whitney U test. A two-sided p-value of <0.05 was considered significant.

Sample size analysis was based on the values of myocardial global work index, suggesting that a sample size of 49 patients will allow sufficient power (β = 0.2) to detect difference from the reference population (α = 0.05). However, due to limited recruitment that was dependent on the population- and institution-related factors, it was not possible to meet this sample. Post hoc power analysis suggests 67.6% power of the present analysis.

3. Results

3.1. Baseline Patient Characteristics

The enrolled patients were mostly middle-aged (median of 62 years), with a higher proportion of male patients (58.3%). The median duration of hemodialysis treatment was 4 years, while most patients were dialysed using the arterio-venous fistula (66.7%). The patients suffered from a high comorbidity burden, including arterial hypertension (86.1%), diabetes mellitus (25.0%), and peripheral artery disease (30.5%) (Supplementary Table S1).

3.2. Comparison of Baseline Echocardiographic Measurements with Reference Values

When analyzing the left ventricular myocardial work and longitudinal strain parameters, the majority of patients with ESRD showed a deviation from the reference range for global wasted work (median of 179.0 vs. 53.0–122.2 mmHg% as reference range), global work efficiency (median of 90.0 vs. 94.0–97.0% as reference range), and average global peak longitudinal strain (median of −16.0 vs. −24.0–(−16.0)% as reference range) (Figure 1 and Supplementary Table S2). There was no deviation for the global work index and global constructed work (Figure 1 and Supplementary Table S2).

To further evaluate the sample data distribution, the 95%CI were determined for the main left ventricular myocardial work and longitudinal strain parameters. This additional analysis suggested consistent findings suggesting that the true measured values of global wasted work and global work efficiency in ESRD patients will, 95% of the time, be outside of the reference ranges (global wasted work: 95%CI of 152.0–223.2 vs. 53.0–122.2 mmHg% as reference range; global work efficiency: 95%CI of 87.2–91.6 vs. 94.0–97.0% as reference range). This was not confirmed for other parameters such as the global work index, global constructed work, and global longitudinal strain (Supplementary Figure S2).

When evaluating the left atrial and ventricular 2D volumes, linear dimensions, and ejection fraction parameters, patients with ESRD showed a deviation from reference range for the left atrial diameter (median of 39.0 vs. 29.3–37.9 mm as reference range), left ventricular end-diastolic indexed volume (median of 114.3 vs. 40.0–62.8 mL/m^2 as reference range), left ventricular end-systolic indexed volume (median of 55.7 vs. 13.4–23.8 mL/m^2 as reference range), left ventricular ejection fraction (median of 57.0 vs. 59.0–68.8% as reference range), left ventricular mass (median of 240.4 vs. 89.4–164.2 g as reference range), and indexed left ventricular mass (median of 122.9 vs. 52.4–87.4 g/m^2 as reference range) (Table 1).

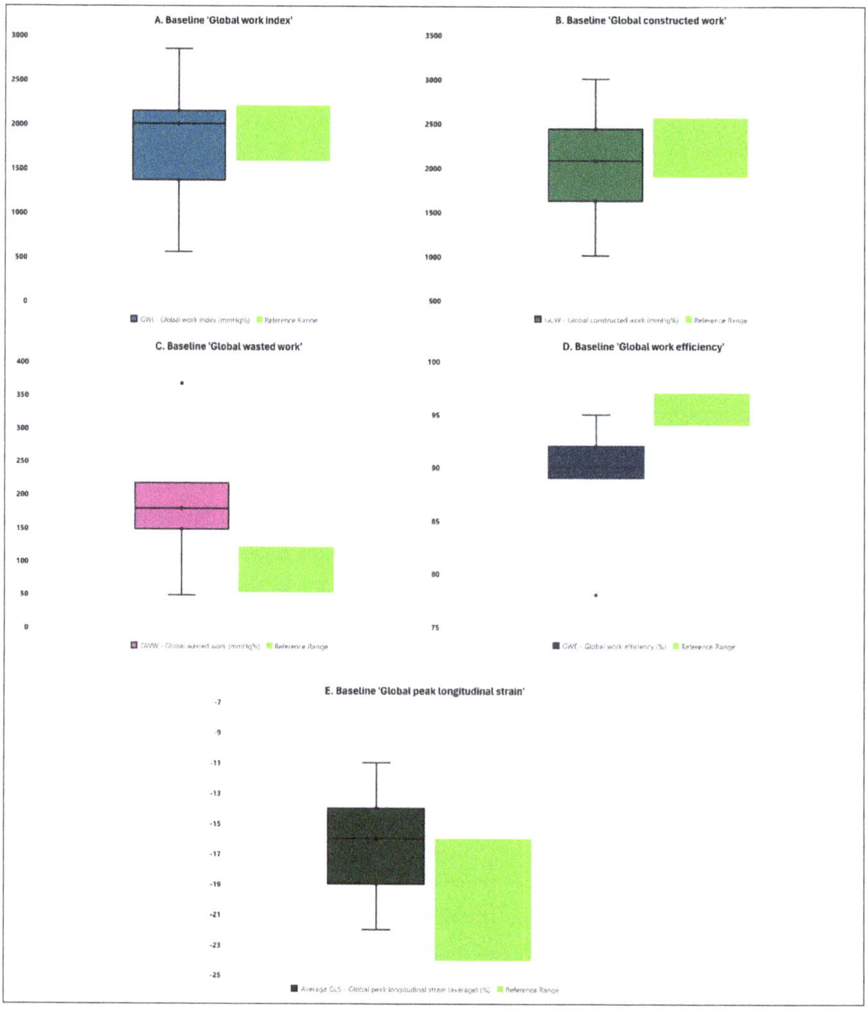

Figure 1. Comparison of baseline contemporary echocardiographic measures of left ventricular myocardial work and longitudinal strain to reference values from the general population (boxes and whiskers plots). Data are presented as boxes and whiskers (median (interquartile range) and minimum/maximum).

Table 1. Comparison of baseline echocardiographic measures of the left atrial and ventricular 2D volumes, linear dimensions, and ejection fraction to reference values from the general population.

Echocardiographic Parameters	Study Sample (Baseline—Hemodialysis Treatment)	Reference Values
LAd—Left atrial diameter (mm)	39.0 (35.0–42.0) *	29.3–37.9
LAVi—Left atrial volume indexed (mL/m^2)	26.0 (19.3–28.15)	18.0–31.6
LVEDV BiP—Left ventricular end-diastolic volume [bi-plane] (mL)	92.5 (67.0–106.0)	68.0–117.6
LVESV BiP—Left ventricular end-systolic volume [bi-plane] (mL)	41.2 (25.0–48.0)	22.8–44.6
LVEF BiP—Left ventricular ejection fraction [bi-plane] (%)	57.0 (53.0–63.0)	59.0–68.8

Table 1. *Cont.*

Echocardiographic Parameters	Study Sample (Baseline—Hemodialysis Treatment)	Reference Values
LVEDVi—Left ventricular end-diastolic volume indexed (mL/m^2)	114.3 (84.0–125.0) *	40.0–62.8
LVESVi—Left ventricular end-systolic volume indexed (mL/m^2)	55.7 (37.0–69.0) *	13.4–23.8
IVSd—Interventricular septal wall thickness (mm)	10.0 (9.0–11.0)	7.0–10.2
LVPWd—Left ventricular posterior wall thickness (mm)	11.0 (10.0–11.0)	7.3–10.3
LVIDd—Left ventricular internal end-diastolic diameter (mm)	51.0 (46.0–54.0)	39.5–49.1
LVIDs—Left ventricular internal end-systolic diameter (mm)	33.0 (26.0–38.0)	25.2–34.6
LVM—Left ventricular mass (g)	240.4 (185.1–280.4) *	89.4–164.2
LVMi—Left ventricular mass indexed (g/m^2)	122.9 (90.6–153.9)	52.4–87.4

Data are expressed as median (interquartile range). * Outside of the reference range. Abbreviations: none.

When analyzes the right ventricular size and function parameters, patients with ESRD showed a deviation from the reference range for tricuspid annular plane systolic excursion (median of 12.2 vs. ≥17.0 mm as reference range) and right ventricular fractional area change (median of 36.6 vs. 41.3–58.1% as reference range) (Table 2).

Table 2. Comparison of baseline echocardiographic measures of the right ventricular size and function parameters to reference values from the general population.

Echocardiographic Parameters	Study Sample (Baseline—Hemodialysis Treatment)	Reference Values
RVEDV—Right ventricular end-diastolic volume (mL)	65.0 (53.0–66.0)	65.0–107.0
RVESV—Right ventricular end-systolic volume (mL)	34.4 (29.0–40.0)	18.0–40.0
3D RVEF (%)—3D right ventricular ejection fraction (%)	45.9 (41.8–51.2) *	>45.0
RV Dd base—Right ventricular diastolic diameter—base (mm)	37.1 (32.0–40.0)	28.7–39.7
RV Dd mid—Right ventricular diastolic diameter—mid (mm)	26.7 (23.0–28.0)	22.5–33.5
RV Ld—Right ventricular longitudinal diameter (mm)	63.1 (59.0–67.0)	59.8–75.8
TAPSE—Tricuspid annular plane systolic excursion (mm)	12.2 (9.0–16.0) *	≥17.0
RV FAC—Right ventricular fractional area change (%)	36.6 (31.2–36.6) *	41.3–58.1

Data are expressed as median (interquartile range). * Not within the reference range. Abbreviations: none.

When analyzing the left ventricular diastolic function and Doppler parameters, patients with ESRD showed a deviation from the reference range for transmitral E wave velocity (median of 80.0 vs. <50.0 cm/s as reference range) and mitral valve deceleration time (median of 291.0 vs. 160.0–220.0 ms as reference range) (Table 3).

Table 3. Comparison of baseline echocardiographic measures of diastolic function and Doppler parameters to reference values from the general population.

Echocardiographic Parameters	Study Sample (Baseline—Hemodialysis Treatment)	Reference Values
MV E vel—Transmitral E wave velocity (cm/s)	80.0 (70.0–100.0) *	<50.0
MV DecT—Mitral valve deceleration time (ms)	291.0 (257.0–356.0) *	160.0–220.0
MV E/A Ratio—Mitral valve E/A Ratio	0.8 (0.6–1.0)	0.8–2.0
e′ Sept—Septal annular e′ velocity (cm/s)	9.8 (5.2–11.3)	>7.0
e′ lat—Lateral annular e′ velocity (cm/s)	10.1 (8.5–11.8)	>10.0
E/e′ average ratio	10.8 (8.7–12.6)	<14.0
PV AccT—Pulmonic valve acceleration time (ms)	155.0 (135.0–166.0)	>120.0
TV S′—Peak systolic tissue velocity (S′ wave) at the tricuspid annulus (cm/s)	10.0 (9.3–11.2)	>9.5

Data are expressed as median (interquartile range). * Not within the reference range. Abbreviations: none.

3.3. Echocardiographic Parameters Following the Hemodialysis-to-Hemodiafiltration Transfer

Following the hemodialysis-to-hemodiafiltration transfer, there was no statistically significant change in the left ventricular myocardial work and longitudinal strain parameters, except in global wasted work that increased (179.0 vs. 233.5 mmHg%, $p = 0.037$), aortic valve opening time that decreased (94.0 vs. 70.0 ms, $p = 0.038$), and mid-inferior peak systolic longitudinal strain that improved (−17.0 vs. −18.7%, $p = 0.016$) at 3-month follow-up (Table 4).

Table 4. Comparison of contemporary echocardiographic measures of left ventricular myocardial work and longitudinal strain following the hemodialysis-to-hemodiafiltration transfer.

Echocardiographic Parameters	Baseline (Hemodialysis Treatment)	3-Month Follow-Up (Hemodiafiltration Treatment)	*p*-Value
GWI—Global work index (mmHg%)	2001.0 (1368.0–2148.0)	1897.5 (1669.0–2396.0)	0.637
GCW—Global constructed work (mmHg%)	2084.5 (1628.0–2440.0)	1939.5 (1793.0–2387.0)	0.886
GWW—Global wasted work (mmHg%)	179.0 (148.0–217.0)	233.5 (159.0–315.0)	0.037
GWE—Global work efficiency (%)	90.0 (89.0–92.0)	89.0 (87.0–91.0)	0.250
AVO—Aortic valve opening (ms)	94.0 (63.0–115.7)	70.0 (50.0–93.0)	0.038
AVC—Aortic valve closure (ms)	361.0 (298.0–384.0)	347.0 (330.0–371.0)	0.422
MVO—Mitral valve opening (ms)	449.7 (411.0–483.0)	453.6 (424.0–471.0)	0.817
MVC—Mitral valve closure (ms)	329.0 (19.0–674.0)	706.0 (53.0–849.0)	0.063
Longitudinal peak strain dispersion (ms)	64.0 (51.0–70.0)	58.1 (51.0–65.0)	0.385
APLAX GLS—Global peak longitudinal strain [APLAX] (%)	−16.0 (−18.0–[−14.0])	−17.1 (−18.0–[−16.0])	0.293
A4C GSL (A4C)—Global peak longitudinal strain [A4C] (%)	−16.0 (−19.0–[−14.0])	−17.0 (−18.0–[−16.0])	0.376
A2C GLS (A2C)—Global peak longitudinal strain [A2C] (%)	−18.0 (−20.0–[−14.0])	−18.2 (−20.0–[−17.0])	0.440
Average GLS—Global peak longitudinal strain (average) (%)	−16.0 (−19.0–[−14.0])	−17.5 (−19.0–[−17.0])	0.258
BA PSSL Full (%)—Basal anterior peak systolic longitudinal strain (%)	−13.8 (−18.0–[−9.0])	−15.0 (−16.0–[−12.0])	0.516
BI PSSL Full (%)—Basal inferior peak systolic longitudinal strain (%)	−15.0 (−17.0–[−10.0])	−15.8 (−18.0–[−14.0])	0.117
MA PSSL Full (%)—Mid-anterior peak systolic longitudinal strain (%)	−15.0 (−19.0–[−9.0])	−15.0 (−18.0–[−13.0])	0.826
MI PSSL Full (%)—Mid-inferior peak systolic longitudinal strain (%)	−17.0 (−19.0–[−11.0])	−18.7 (−20.0–[−18.0])	0.016
AA PSSL Full (%)—Apical anterior peak systolic longitudinal strain (%)	−21.0 (−29.0–[−18.0])	−21.0 (−24.0–[−17.0])	0.590
AI PSSL Full (%)—Apical inferior peak systolic longitudinal strain (%)	−22.0 (−32.0–[−18.0])	−25.5 (−31.0–[−23.0])	0.379
BAS PSSL Full (%)—Basal anteroseptal peak systolic longitudinal strain (%)	−12.0 (−14.0–[−8.0])	−13.0 (−16.0––10.0])	0.107
BP PSSL Full (%)—Basal posterior peak systolic longitudinal strain (%)	−14.0 (−18.0–[−10.0])	−15.3 (−17.0–[−12.0])	0.467
MAS PSSL Full (%)—Mid-anteroseptal peak systolic longitudinal strain (%)	−20.0 (−23.0–[−15.0])	−20.1 (−23.0–[−18.0])	0.441
MP PSSL Full (%)—Mid-posterior peak systolic longitudinal strain (%)	−17.0 (−19.0–[−13.0])	−16.1 (−19.0–[−12.0])	0.930
AS PSSL Full (%)—Apico-anteroseptal peak systolic longitudinal strain (%)	−24.0 (−29.0––14.0])	−23.0 (−27.0–[−21.0])	0.733
AP PSSL Full (%)—Apical posterior peak systolic longitudinal strain (%)	−20.0 (−28.0–[−14.0])	−18.3 (−20.0–[−16.0])	0.590
BS PSSL Full (%)—Basal septal peak systolic longitudinal strain (%)	−11.0 (−15.0–[−6.0])	−11.7 (−13.0–[−10.0])	0.567
BL PSSL Full (%)—Basal lateral peak systolic longitudinal strain (%)	−13.0 (−17.0–[−11.0])	−14.0 (−17.0–[−12.0])	0.800

Table 4. *Cont.*

Echocardiographic Parameters	Baseline (Hemodialysis Treatment)	3-Month Follow-Up (Hemodiafiltration Treatment)	p-Value
MS PSSL Full (%)—Mid-septal peak systolic longitudinal strain (%)	−18.0 (−21.0–[−14.0])	−19.0 (−21.0–[−17.0])	0.454
ML PSSL Full (%)—Mid-lateral peak systolic longitudinal strain (%)	−17.0 (−19.0–[−12.0])	−16.6 (−19.0–[−14.0])	0.692
AS PSSL Full (%)—Apical septal peak systolic longitudinal strain (%)	−23.0 (−29.0–[−16.0])	−23.0 (−26.0–[−21.0])	0.912
AL PSSL Full (%)—Apical lateral peak systolic longitudinal strain (%)	−21.0 (−27.0–[−12.0])	−18.5 (−23.0–[−14.0])	0.545

Data are expressed as median (interquartile range) and compared using the Mann–Whitney U test. Abbreviations: none.

Furthermore, there was no statistically significant change in the left atrial and ventricular 2D volumes, linear dimensions, and ejection fraction parameters, except in interventricular septal diameter that decreased (10.0 vs. 9.0 mm, $p = 0.013$), left ventricular posterior wall diastolic diameter that decreased (11.0 vs. 9.0 mm, $p = 0.004$), and left ventricular posterior wall systolic diameter that decreased (14.0 vs. 13.0 mm, $p = 0.028$) at 3-month follow-up (Table 5).

Table 5. Comparison of contemporary echocardiographic measures of left atrial and ventricular 2D volumes, linear dimensions, and ejection fraction following the hemodialysis-to-hemodiafiltration transfer.

Echocardiographic Parameters	Baseline (Hemodialysis Treatment)	3-Month Follow-Up (Hemodiafiltration Treatment)	p-Value
Left atrium			
LALs A2C—Left atrial length—systolic [A2C] (mm)	53.0 (41.0–57.0)	54.0 (48.0–59.0)	0.190
LAESV A-L A2C—Left atrial end-systolic volume, area-length [A2C] (mL)	49.0 (32.0–68.0)	52.0 (45.0–71.0)	0.333
LAESV MOD A2C—Left atrial end-systolic volume, method of discs [A2C] (mL)	47.0 (31.0–67.0)	54.0 (42.0–68.0)	0.291
LALs A4C—Left atrial length—systolic [A4C] (mm)	56.0 (50.0–62.0)	56.0 (54.0–62.0)	0.620
LAESV A-L A4C—Left atrial end-systolic volume, area-length [A4C] (mL)	44.5 (35.0–60.0)	52.0 (43.0–57.0)	0.692
LAESV MOD A4C—Left atrial end-systolic volume, method of discs [A4C] (mL)	44.0 (33.0–60.0)	51.0 (40.0–58.0)	0.590
LAESV AL—Left atrial end-systolic volume, area-length [derived] (mL)	51.0 (39.0–65.0)	55.0 (45.0–61.0)	0.409
LAVi—Left atrial volume indexed (mL/m^2)	26.0 (19.3–28.15)	28.1 (23.5–30.6)	0.214
Left ventricle			
LVVED 4Ch—Left ventricular end-diastolic volume [4Ch] (mL)	76.0 (59.0–103.0)	77.3 (68.0–84.0)	0.826
LVVES 4Ch—Left ventricular end-systolic volume [4Ch] (mL)	32.0 (20.0–44.0)	36.4 (30.0–45.0)	0.575
LVEF 4Ch—Left ventricular ejection fraction [4Ch] (%)	57.2 (50.0–66.0)	53.1 (51.0–56.0)	0.153
LVSV 4Ch—Left ventricular stroke volume [4Ch] (mL)	42.0 (39.0–53.0)	40.8 (28.0–47.0)	0.190
LVCO 4Ch—Left ventricular cardiac output [4Ch] (L/min)	3.6 (2.6–4.1)	(2.8–3.4)	0.053
LVLs 4Ch—Left ventricular length in systole [4Ch] (mm)	61.0 (55.0–66.0)	61.0 (58.0–67.0)	0.523
LVLd 4Ch—Left ventricular length in diastole [4Ch] (mm)	72.0 (67.0–77.0)	73.0 (72.0–77.0)	0.461

Table 5. *Cont.*

Echocardiographic Parameters	Baseline (Hemodialysis Treatment)	3-Month Follow-Up (Hemodiafiltration Treatment)	*p*-Value
LVVED 2Ch—Left ventricular end-diastolic volume [2Ch] (mL)	89.0 (56.0–107.0)	85.0 (74.0–90.0)	0.982
LVVES 2Ch—Left ventricular end-systolic volume [2Ch] (mL)	32.0 (24.0–48.0)	35.3 (27.0–40.0)	0.886
LVEF 2Ch—Left ventricular ejection fraction [2Ch] (%)	57.0 (54.0–60.0)	60.2 (57.0–52.0)	0.088
LVSV 2Ch—Left ventricular stroke volume [2Ch] (mL)	47.0 (35.0–61.0)	51.0 (42.0–55.0)	0.410
LVCO 2Ch—Left ventricular cardiac output [2Ch] (L/min)	3.4 (2.5–4.3)	3.5 (3.1–3.8)	0.676
LVLs 2Ch—Left ventricular length in systole [2Ch] (mm)	6.3 (5.7–6.9)	6.4 (5.9–6.7)	0.582
LVLs 2Ch—Left ventricular length in diastole [2Ch] (mm)	7.4 (6.6–8.0)	7.7 (7.1–8.1)	0.317
LVVED BiP—Left ventricular end-diastolic volume [biplane] (mL)	92.5 (67.0–106.0)	82.8 (72.0–97.0)	0.367
LVVES BiP—Left ventricular end-systolic volume [biplane] (mL)	41.2 (25.0–48.0)	36.6 (30.0–39.0)	0.488
LVEF BiP -Left ventricular ejection fraction [biplane] (%)	57.0 (53.0–63.0)	56.5 (55.0–60.0)	0.644
LVSV BiP—Left ventricular stroke volume [biplane] (mL)	49.0 (38.0–58.0)	46.2 (42.0–29.0)	0.530
LVCO BiP—Left ventricular cardiac output [biplane] (L/min)	3.7 (3.0–4.0)	3.2 (3.0–3.4)	0.052
LVVED 4D—Left ventricular end-diastolic volume [4-dimensional] (mL)	114.3 (84.0 –125.0)	103.6 (73.0–122.0)	0.404
LVVES 4D—Left ventricular end-systolic volume [4-dimensional] (mL)	55.7 (37.0–69.0)	46.9 (34.0–54.0)	0.126
CO 4D—Cardiac output [4-dimensional] (L/min)	4.0 (3.2–4.5)	3.7 (2.9–4.6)	0.344
Spl—Sphericity index	0.4 (0.3–0.5)	0.4 (0.3–0.5)	0.455
IVSd—Interventricular septal thickness in diastole (mm)	10.0 (9.0–11.0)	9.0 (8.0–10.0)	0.013
LVIDd—Left ventricular internal end-diastolic diameter (mm)	51.0 (46.0–54.0)	51.0 (48.0–55.0)	0.860
LVPWd—Left ventricular posterior wall thickness in diastole (mm)	11.0 (10.0–11.0)	9.0 (8.0–10.0)	0.004
IVSs—Interventricular septal thickness in systole (mm)	13.0 (11.0–14.0)	12.0 (11.0–13.0)	0.062
LVIDs—Left ventricular internal end-systolic diameter (mm)	33.0 (26.0–38.0)	33.0 (31.0–36.0)	0.461
LVPWs—Left ventricular posterior wall thickness in systole (mm)	14.0 (13.0–15.0)	13.0 (12.0–14.0)	0.028
EDV Teich—Left ventricular end-diastolic volume [Teicholz] (mL)	127.1 (96.0–140.0)	127.0 (105.0–147.0)	0.904
ESV Teich—Left ventricular end-systolic volume [Teicholz] (mL)	46.9 (24.0–61.0)	47.0 (38.0–54.0)	0.538
LVEF Teich—Left ventricular ejection fraction [Teicholz] (%)	64.6 (59.0–73.0)	63.1 (61.0–66.0)	0.553
%FS—Left ventricular fractional shortening (%)	36.0 (32.0–42.0)	35.0 (33.0–37.0)	0.434
LVSV Teich—Left ventricular stroke volume [Teicholz] (mL)	80.0 (57.0–107.0)	79.0 (68.0–93.0)	0.965
LVd Mass—Left ventricular mass (g)	240.4 (185.1–280.4)	211.4 (165.1–258.0)	0.150
LVMi—Left ventricular mass indexed (g/m^2)	122.9 (90.6–153.9)	103.6 (81.6–155.5)	0.123
Ao diam—Aortic diameter (mm)	33.0 (30.0–36.0)	32.0 (30.0–35.0)	0.620

Table 5. *Cont.*

Echocardiographic Parameters	Baseline (Hemodialysis Treatment)	3-Month Follow-Up (Hemodiafiltration Treatment)	p-Value
LA diam—Left atrial diameter (mm)	39.0 (35.0–42.0)	40.0 (37.0–43.0)	0.628
LA/Ao—Left atrium/aorta ratio	1.2 (1.1–1.2)	1.2 (1.1–1.4)	0.129

Data are expressed as median (interquartile range) and compared using the Mann–Whitney U test. Abbreviations: none.

When evaluating the left ventricular diastolic function and Doppler parameters, there was no statistically significant change following the hemodialysis-to-hemodiafiltration transfer (Table 6).

Table 6. Comparison of contemporary echocardiographic measures of left ventricular diastolic function and Doppler parameters following the hemodialysis-to-hemodiafiltration transfer.

Echocardiographic Parameters	Baseline (Hemodialysis Treatment)	3-Month Follow-Up (Hemodiafiltration Treatment)	p-Value
MV E vel—Mitral valve E wave velocity (m/s)	0.8 (0.7–1.0)	0.9 (0.7–1.0)	0.397
MV DecT—Mitral valve deceleration time (ms)	291.0 (257.0–356.0)	306.5 (244.0–346.0)	0.660
MV Dec Slope—Mitral valve deceleration slope (m/s^2)	2.8 (2.1–3.4)	3.3 (2.3–3.7)	0.361
MV A Vel—Mitral valve A wave velocity (m/s)	1.0 (0.8–1.1)	1.0 (0.9–1.2)	0.428
MV E/A Ratio—Mitral valve E/A wave ratio	0.8 (0.6–1.0)	0.9 (0.7–1.0)	0.397
Average septal annular e′ velocity (cm/s)	9.8 (5.2–11.3)	9.6 (5.3–10.9)	0.190
E/e′ Sept—E to e′ wave ratio at septal mitral annulus	13.4 (11.2–15.7)	13.7 (11.8–15.6)	0.982
Average lateral annular e′ velocity (cm/s)	10.1 (8.5–11.8)	9.7 (8.4–11.3)	0.525
E/e′ Lat—E to e′ wave ratio at lateral mitral annulus	8.9 (7.0–10.4)	9.3 (8.0–9.6)	0.613
E/e′ Avg—E/e′ average ratio	10.8 (8.7–12.6)	11.1 (9.7–11.3)	0.939
AV Vmax—Aortic valve maximal velocity (m/s)	1.5 (1.2–1.8)	1.6 (1.3–1.7)	0.403
AV Vmean—Aortic valve mean velocity (m/s)	1.2 (0.8–1.3)	1.1 (0.9–1.1)	0.684
AV maxPG—Aortic valve maximal pressure gradient (mmHg)	10.6 (6.7–12.6)	11.2 (7.2–11.9)	0.921
AV meanPG—Aortic valve mean pressure gradient (mmHg)	6.4 (3.1–7.0)	6.2 (4.0–6.4)	0.809
AV Env. Ti—Aortic valve envelope time (ms)	313.5 (262.0–352.0)	310.7 (304.0–343.0)	0.636
AV VTI—Aortic valve velocity-time integral (cm)	33.1 (26.5–35.3)	36.6 (30.0–36.8)	0.146
PV AccT—Pulmonic valve acceleration time (ms)	155.0 (135.0–166.0)	151.0 (138.0–156.0)	0.684
PV Acc Slope—Pulmonic valve acceleration slope (m/s^2)	5.9 (4.8–6.9)	6.2 (5.0–6.7)	0.947
Peak systolic tissue velocity (S′ wave) at the tricuspid annulus (cm/s)	10.0 (9.3–11.2)	10.4 (9.1–12.2)	0.273

Data are expressed as median (interquartile range) and compared using the Mann–Whitney U test. Abbreviations: none.

Finally, there was no statistically significant change in the right ventricular size and function parameters, except in the right ventricular diastolic diameter at mid-ventricle that increased (26.7 vs. 28.9 mm, $p = 0.042$) following the hemodialysis-to-hemodiafiltration transfer (Table 7).

Table 7. Comparison of contemporary echocardiographic measures of right ventricular size and function parameters following the hemodialysis-to-hemodiafiltration transfer.

Echocardiographic Parameters	Baseline (Hemodialysis Treatment)	3-Month Follow-Up (Hemodiafiltration Treatment)	*p*-Value
RVEDV—Right ventricular end-diastolic volume (mL)	65.0 (53.0–66.0)	59.9 (47.0–68.0)	0.361
RVESV—Right ventricular end-systolic volume (mL)	34.4 (29.0–40.0)	32.5 (29.0–35.0)	0.305
3D RVEF (%)—3D right ventricular ejection fraction (%)	45.9 (41.8–51.2)	45.9 (38.2–48.6)	0.434
RV SV—Right ventricular stroke volume (mL)	29.9 (24.0–33.0)	27.7 (21.0–32.0)	0.494
RV Dd base—Right ventricular diastolic diameter—base (mm)	37.1 (32.0–40.0)	35.6 (34.0–37.0)	0.152
RV Dd mid—Right ventricular diastolic diameter—mid (mm)	26.7 (23.0–28.0)	28.9 (27.0–31.0)	0.042
RVLd—Right ventricular longitudinal diameter (mm)	63.1 (59.0–67.0)	60.5 (58.0–61.0)	0.134
TAPSE—Tricuspid annular plane systolic excursion (mm)	12.2 (9.0–16.0)	12.4 (10.0–14.0)	0.886
RV FAC—Right ventricular fractional area change (%)	36.6 (31.2–36.6)	39.5 (31.0–42.4)	0.182

Data are expressed as median (interquartile range) and compared using the Mann–Whitney U test. Abbreviations: none.

3.4. *Evaluation of the Laboratory Parameters and the Efficacy of Dialysis during the 3-Month Follow-Up*

There was no statistically significant difference in the main laboratory parameters following the hemodialysis-to-hemodiafiltration transfer, except in hemoglobin levels that decreased at 3-month follow-up (119.0 vs. 109.0 g/L, $p = 0.009$) (Supplementary Table S3).

Following the hemodialysis-to-hemodiafiltration transfer, there was a significant decrease in the levels of β2 microglobulin (46.8 vs. 9.6 mg/L, $p < 0.001$) and a statistically significant increase in the Kt/V ratio (1.2 vs. 1.4, $p = 0.024$), indicating a higher efficacy of dialysis treatment with hemodiafiltration (Supplementary Table S4).

4. Discussion

This study provides important data about contemporary echocardiographic measures in patients with ESRD undergoing hemodialysis-to-hemodiafiltration transfer. To the best of our knowledge, there are no studies evaluating the myocardial work and strain in patients undergoing hemodialysis-to-hemodiafiltration transfer. Several prior studies compared the conventional echocardiographic measures between patients receiving conventional hemodialysis and those receiving on-line hemodiafiltration [7,26–29]. Furthermore, few studies evaluated contemporary echocardiographic measures solely in patients receiving conventional hemodialysis [30–33], but not concerning transfer to hemodiafiltration. The comprehensive assessment of contemporary echocardiographic parameters in ESRD patients, both at baseline and during the transition between dialysis techniques, could contribute to our understanding of cardiac dynamics in this population. An additional purpose of this underpowered study is its hypothesis-generating potential for future research on advanced cardiovascular imaging in patients with terminal renal disease. It may also stimulate further research and the development of novel non-invasive cardiovascular diagnostic and therapeutic modalities in this population.

There are several main findings of this study. First, patients with ESRD showed baseline deviations of global wasted work, global work efficiency, and average global peak longitudinal strain, suggesting an impaired myocardial work and strain function compared to the general population. Second, patients with ESRD exhibited significantly higher left atrial diameters, left ventricular volumes, and left ventricular mass compared to the general population, which is consistent with chronic volume/pressure overloading. Third, the raw measures of left ventricular (ejection fraction) and right ventricular systolic function (tricuspid annular plane systolic excursion and fractional area change) were impaired in ESRD patients suggesting the biventricular affection in this population. Finally, following the hemodialysis-to-hemodiafiltration transfer, there was no significant change in most contemporary and conventional echocardiographic measures, except for an increase in global wasted work.

Hemodiafiltration has been associated with better cardiovascular outcomes compared to hemodialysis [1,7,8,34], but objective methods of cardiovascular assessment are lacking. There is evidence that hemodiafiltration is associated with a better hemodynamic balance with less intradialytic hypotension, better blood pressure control, and more stable endothelial function [1]. Additionally, a more effective removal of middle-weight molecules, such as β2-microglobulin, may mitigate myocardial hypertrophy in this population. Takayama et al. published a high proportion of amyloid fibrils in the myocardium of long-term chronic maintenance hemodialysis patients [35]. Hypothetically, a better removal of other middle-weight molecules such as cytokines, advanced glycation end products, pentraxin-3, visfatin, adiponectin, leptin, and fibroblast growth factors could be associated with slower progressive atherosclerosis and valve calcification and therefore can slow down the progression of coronary artery disease and valve disease [9].

The speckle-tracking-derived global longitudinal strain emerged as an important contemporary echocardiographic parameter for the early detection of left ventricular dysfunction [36]. Several studies showed its relevance in detecting subclinical myocardial dysfunction amongst patients receiving conventional hemodialysis, particularly in those with a preserved ejection fraction [5,15,30,31,37]. These studies suggest that global longitudinal strain outperforms ejection fraction in predicting both all-cause and cardiovascular mortality, emphasizing its importance in this specific patient group [14]. Previous studies have also shown an association of impaired global longitudinal strain with impaired prognosis in this population [12,13]. The present study showed lower values of global longitudinal strain in hemodialysis patients, when compared to established reference intervals, suggesting the presence of left ventricular dysfunction in this population. This is consistent with previous studies comparing ESRD patients and the general population [30,31,33,38]. However, due to the specific characteristics of ESRD patients and their unique pathophysiology, there are potential biases in using general population values as a reference. Specifically, ESRD patients have inherently increased cardiac loading conditions and frequently exhibit humoral disbalance that may lead to microvascular dysfunction, cardiomyocyte impairments, and electrolyte-related channelopathies. Therefore, it is unclear if ESRD patients require different cut-off values for contemporary echocardiographic measures, and careful interpretation of these findings is mandatory.

Another contemporary echocardiographic measure of significance is myocardial work, which has emerged as a novel and sensitive parameter for evaluating systolic function. Despite not being widely incorporated into everyday clinical practice, myocardial work has the potential for broader utilization due to its ability to consider dynamic cardiac contraction in various loading circumstances and afterload-dependent restrictions [17]. There is growing interest in exploring the applicability of myocardial work in assessing left ventricular function in patients undergoing chronic maintenance hemodialysis [39]. The present study revealed that hemodialysis patients exhibit a significantly impaired 'myocardial work' function, including a decreased GWE and increased GWW, compared to established reference intervals. This is consistent with a recent study showing significantly reduced GWE in patients undergoing chronic maintenance hemodialysis, but there was no significant difference in left ventricular ejection fraction [40], which is contrary to the findings from this analysis. This disagreement may be associated with a difference in hemodialysis efficiency, or due to differences in the reference population (age- and sex matched controls subjects vs. reference values from the general population) [40]. Further research in this area is therefore warranted to establish the potential clinical applications and implications of myocardial work measurements in the ESRD population.

A crucial aspect of the study involved comparing contemporary echocardiographic measurements with subsequent control findings post-hemodialysis-to-hemodiafiltration transfer. A transfer to hemodiafiltration may be associated with positive cardiovascular effects [1,7–10], and there are several potential mechanistic hemodynamic effects of hemodiafiltration versus hemodialysis that could mediate differences in the myocardial work indices [29,32,33]. Firstly, hemodiafiltration should include more gradual and controlled fluid removal due to its combination of diffusion and convection, thereby avoiding significant oscillations of autonomous nervous system and peripheral vascular resistance (afterload) [29]. Secondly, controlled fluid removal with hemodiafiltration may prevent sudden shifts in intravascular volume, thereby maintaining a more stable preload. Thirdly, hemodiafiltration may have more favourable effects on the myocardial work indices by avoiding sudden changes in cardiac loading conditions, which translate to increased myocardial oxygen demand [32,33]. Nevertheless, this analysis did not show significant difference in most parameters of the global longitudinal strain and myocardial work, except for the mid-inferior peak systolic longitudinal strain that improved following the transfer, coupled with an increase in global wasted work. The observed beneficial changes in segmental longitudinal strain could represent an early echocardiographic sign of hemodynamic effects of hemodiafiltration. However, the unchanged global longitudinal strain and paradoxically increased global wasted work may reflect more complex associations in vivo. Firstly, global longitudinal strain is sensitive to an increased wall stress [31], which is not necessarily resolved with hemodiafiltration. Despite theoretically more effective and gradual volume reduction with hemodiafiltration, the variability of sympathetic activation, and compensatory increase in arterial afterload is unpredictable, thereby potentially promoting an increase in global wasted work. Secondly, this study did not account for the measures of cardiac electromechanical synchrony such as the presence of bundle branch blocks, which may affect the global wasted work [20] and may bias the observed findings. Fourthly, cardiac remodelling may require more time than the scheduled post-transfer follow-up. Finally, the underpowered sample size of the study could hamper the differentiation of any statistical difference between the time points. Future powered studies are therefore needed to detect the underlying trends and mechanisms of the interaction between hemodiafiltration and myocardial work/strain in ESRD patients. The current body of literature does not contain any study investigating contemporary echocardiographic measures concerning hemodialysis-to-hemodiafiltration transfer.

The commonly utilized conventional measures of left and right ventricular systolic function were found to be impaired in hemodialysis patients in this study, a finding consistent with previous research [32,41]. This indicates a biventricular dysfunction within this patient population, likely attributable to a combination of volume and pressure overload, along with latent ischemia caused by microcirculatory dysfunction resulting from hemodynamic oscillations in myocardial perfusion during hemodialysis sessions [5]. Additionally, the direct impact of uremia may further contribute to the observed myocardial impairment. This study also observed a high proportion of left ventricular hypertrophy, volume enlargement, and increased mass—all recognized as robust predictors of cardiovascular mortality. These conditions, often associated with both high-volume overload and pressure overload, have been consistently reported in prior studies [42,43]. These findings underscore the intricate relationship between hemodialysis and adverse cardiac remodelling, emphasizing the need for targeted interventions to mitigate the heightened cardiovascular risks in this patient cohort.

Several studies investigated the conventional echocardiographic parameters, such as the left ventricular ejection fraction and mass, in distinct patient groups receiving different hemodialysis types [7,26,28,29]. Studies comparing the hemodialysis and hemodiafiltration cohorts revealed a significant increase in ejection fraction following the treatment initiation in the hemodiafiltration cohort, but not in those treated with hemodialysis [28,44]. Similarly, the beneficial effects of hemodiafiltration on the regression of left ventricular mass were previously reported [7,45]. However, the available literature reports are inconsistent, with meta-analysis suggesting no significant association of left ventricular ejection fraction and mass between patients receiving hemodialysis and hemodiafiltration treatment [26,29]. This is consistent with the present study, showing no difference in left ventricular ejection fraction and mass following the hemodialysis-to-hemodiafiltration transfer in a single patient group. Therefore, the pathophysiology of left ventricular hypertrophy and impairment may be multifactorial and not necessarily related to the treatment received.

This study has several noteworthy limitations that merit emphasis. Firstly, the limited sample size poses a constraint on the power of the analysis and the generalizability of the findings. Secondly, the inclusion of single time point during the follow-up within a relatively short period hampers the ability to monitor the dynamics of changes and draw inferences about long-term follow-up data. Thirdly, it is crucial to acknowledge the presence of confounding variables, particularly concerning the possibility of subclinical cardiovascular events that could impact myocardial function, thereby influencing echocardiographic findings. Fourthly, it is essential to recognize that echocardiography, being an operator-dependent technique, may introduce potential deviations in measurements. Specifically, despite eliminating the bias of inter-observer variability by focusing on only one experienced echocardiographer, this analysis contained a residual bias of intra-observer variability and bias of within-subject variability. Fifthly, a comparison with sex- and age-matched controls without renal disease would be more appropriate than a comparison with reference values. Also, parallel evaluation of echocardiographic changes in with patients continuing standard haemodialysis may add some additional benefit to the study. Furthermore, this study shares inherent limitations common to observational research. Finally, the parameters of volume status, such as bioimpedance, lung ultrasound, inferior vena cava diameter, interdialytic weight changes, and ultrafiltration per dialysis session, were not monitored for this study. Consequently, the potential effects of these parameters on echocardiographic measurements could not be thoroughly evaluated, introducing a limitation in the comprehensiveness and depth of the analysis.

There are several clinical and scientific implications of this study. Firstly, it provides novel data suggesting impaired contemporary echocardiographic measures such as global longitudinal strain and myocardial work in hemodialysis patients. Having in mind an association of these parameters with cardiovascular prognosis [11–14], this study may urge clinicians for routine and early advanced echocardiographic referral in this population. An early detection of subtle cardiac impairment by advanced echocardiography may help in risk stratification and the timely detection of patients at risk. This information may translate into closer clinical follow-up, stronger preventive measures, stringent lipid lowering, and modifications of renal replacement therapy. Increased clinician's awareness may improve the cardiovascular risk reduction by strict blood pressure control, smoking cessation programmes, or diet modifications. In addition, early prescription of cardioprotective medications, such as sodium–glucose cotransporter inhibitors, which are currently not well investigated in ESRD patients, may gain more attention. Secondly, these findings support the need for routine multidisciplinary team assessment in hemodialysis patients to meet the rising demands of the disease burden. Regular cardiologic counselling for ESRD patients could therefore become the standard of care, particularly in those with subtle echocardiographic impairments, to timely prevent adverse events [11–14]. Finally, this underpowered study has a hypothesis-generating purpose by setting a background for further research in this insufficiently researched area. Future powered studies on this topic may lead to the development of ESRD-specific reference ranges for myocardial work and strain, while future risk stratification tools in ESRD population could incorporate advanced echocardiographic parameters. Hemodiafiltration warrants more scientific attention to clearly delineate whether it truly represents a more favourable dialysis modality from cardiovascular perspective. The development of targeted interventions and monitoring strategies to address the unique cardiovascular challenges faced by individuals with ESRD is prioritized.

5. Conclusions

In conclusion, this study highlights baseline deviations in global wasted work, global work efficiency, and average global peak longitudinal strain among patients with ESRD undergoing hemodialysis, indicative of impaired myocardial work and strain function compared to the general population. Notably, the transition from hemodialysis to hemodiafiltration showed no significant changes in most contemporary echocardiographic measures. These findings warrant further exploration through additional sufficiently powered prospective studies in the field.

Supplementary Materials: The following supporting information can be downloaded at https://www.mdpi.com/article/10.3390/medicina60091537/s1, Supplementary Figure S1. Flow diagram; Supplementary Figure S2. Comparison of baseline contemporary echocardiographic measures of left ventricular myocardial work and longitudinal strain to reference values from the general population (mean and 95% confidence intervals); Supplementary Table S1. Baseline characteristics of the study sample; Supplementary Table S2. Comparison of baseline contemporary echocardiographic measures of left ventricular myocardial work and longitudinal strain to reference values from the general population; Supplementary Table S3. Baseline laboratory parameters of the study sample; Supplementary Table S4. Relevant laboratory measurements regarding the dialysis treatment: pre-dialysis and post-dialysis (at study onset and 3-month follow-up). Supplementary STROBE Statement—checklist of items that should be included in reports of observational studies.

Author Contributions: Conceptualization, J.D.M., A.M. and D.B.K.; methodology, J.D.M., A.M. and J.B.; software, J.D.M. and A.M.; validation, J.D.M., T.D.Š., I.J., J.B. and D.B.Š.; formal analysis, J.D.M., A.M. and J.B.; investigation, J.D.M., I.J. and D.B.K.; resources, J.D.M.; data curation, J.D.M. and T.D.Š.; writing—original draft preparation, J.D.M. and T.D.Š.; writing—review and editing, J.D.M., A.M., D.B.K., I.J., D.B.Š. and J.B.; visualization, J.D.M. and A.M.; supervision, A.M. and J.B.; project administration, J.D.M. All authors have read and agreed to the published version of the manuscript.

Funding: This research received no external funding.

Institutional Review Board Statement: The study was conducted following the Declaration of Helsinki and approved by the Ethics Committee of the University Hospital of Split (No. 2181-147-01/06; date of approval 28 May 2021).

Informed Consent Statement: Informed consent was obtained from all subjects involved in the study.

Data Availability Statement: The datasets used and/or analyzed during the current study are available from the corresponding author on reasonable request.

Conflicts of Interest: The authors declare no conflicts of interest.

References

1. Canaud, B.; Blankestijn, P.J.; Grooteman, M.P.C.; Davenport, A. Why and how high volume hemodiafiltration may reduce cardiovascular mortality in stage 5 chronic kidney disease dialysis patients? A comprehensive literature review on mechanisms involved. *Semin. Dial.* **2022**, *35*, 117–128. [CrossRef] [PubMed]
2. Ma, L.; Zhao, S. Risk factors for mortality in patients undergoing hemodialysis: A systematic review and meta-analysis. *Int. J. Cardiol.* **2017**, *238*, 151–158. [CrossRef] [PubMed]
3. Wang, Z.; Jiang, A.; Wei, F.; Chen, H. Cardiac valve calcification and risk of cardiovascular or all-cause mortality in dialysis patients: A meta-analysis. *BMC Cardiovasc. Disord.* **2018**, *18*, 12. [CrossRef] [PubMed]
4. Assa, S.; Hummel, Y.M.; Voors, A.A.; Kuipers, J.; Westerhuis, R.; de Jong, P.E.; Franssen, C.F.M. Hemodialysis-Induced Regional Left Ventricular Systolic Dysfunction: Prevalence, Patient and Dialysis Treatment-Related Factors, and Prognostic Significance. *Clin. J. Am. Soc. Nephrol.* **2012**, *7*, 1615–1623. [CrossRef] [PubMed]
5. Kott, J.; Reichek, N.; Butler, J.; Arbeit, L.; Mallipattu, S.K. Cardiac Imaging in Dialysis Patients. *Kidney Med.* **2020**, *2*, 629–638. [CrossRef] [PubMed]
6. Burton, J.O.; Jefferies, H.J.; Selby, N.M.; McIntyre, C.W. Hemodialysis-induced cardiac injury: Determinants and associated outcomes. *Clin. J. Am. Soc. Nephrol.* **2009**, *4*, 914–920. [CrossRef]
7. Ohtake, T.; Oka, M.; Ishioka, K.; Honda, K.; Mochida, Y.; Maesato, K.; Moriya, H.; Hidaka, S.; Kobayashi, S. Cardiovascular protective effects of on-line hemodiafiltration: Comparison with conventional hemodialysis. *Ther. Apher. Dial.* **2012**, *16*, 181–188. [CrossRef]
8. Blankestijn, P.J.; Vernooij, R.W.M.; Hockham, C.; Strippoli, G.F.M.; Canaud, B.; Hegbrant, J.; Barth, C.; Covic, A.; Cromm, K.; Cucui, A.; et al. Effect of Hemodiafiltration or Hemodialysis on Mortality in Kidney Failure. *N. Engl. J. Med.* **2023**, *389*, 700–709. [CrossRef]
9. Wolley, M.; Jardine, M.; Hutchison, C.A. Exploring the Clinical Relevance of Providing Increased Removal of Large Middle Molecules. *Clin. J. Am. Soc. Nephrol.* **2018**, *13*, 805–814. [CrossRef]
10. Lang, T.; Zawada, A.M.; Theis, L.; Braun, J.; Ottillinger, B.; Kopperschmidt, P.; Gagel, A.; Kotanko, P.; Stauss-Grabo, M.; Kennedy, J.P.; et al. Hemodiafiltration: Technical and Medical Insights. *Bioengineering* **2023**, *10*, 145. [CrossRef]

11. Hensen, L.C.R.; Goossens, K.; Delgado, V.; Rotmans, J.I.; Jukema, J.W.; Bax, J.J. Prognostic Implications of Left Ventricular Global Longitudinal Strain in Predialysis and Dialysis Patients. *Am. J. Cardiol.* **2017**, *120*, 500–504. [CrossRef]
12. Liu, Y.W.; Su, C.T.; Sung, J.M.; Wang, S.P.; Su, Y.R.; Yang, C.S.; Tsai, L.M.; Chen, J.H.; Tsai, W.C. Association of left ventricular longitudinal strain with mortality among stable hemodialysis patients with preserved left ventricular ejection fraction. *Clin. J. Am. Soc. Nephrol.* **2013**, *8*, 1564–1574. [CrossRef] [PubMed]
13. Kramann, R.; Erpenbeck, J.; Schneider, R.K.; Röhl, A.B.; Hein, M.; Brandenburg, V.M.; van Diepen, M.; Dekker, F.; Marx, N.; Floege, J.; et al. Speckle tracking echocardiography detects uremic cardiomyopathy early and predicts cardiovascular mortality in ESRD. *J. Am. Soc. Nephrol.* **2014**, *25*, 2351–2365. [CrossRef] [PubMed]
14. Krishnasamy, R.; Isbel, N.M.; Hawley, C.M.; Pascoe, E.M.; Burrage, M.; Leano, R.; Haluska, B.A.; Marwick, T.H.; Stanton, T. Left Ventricular Global Longitudinal Strain (GLS) Is a Superior Predictor of All-Cause and Cardiovascular Mortality When Compared to Ejection Fraction in Advanced Chronic Kidney Disease. *PLoS ONE* **2015**, *10*, e0127044. [CrossRef] [PubMed]
15. WHO Consortium. Physical status: The use and interpretation of anthropometry. Report of a WHO Expert Committee. *World Health Organ. Tech. Rep. Ser.* **1995**, *854*, 1–452.
16. Galderisi, M.; Cosyns, B.; Edvardsen, T.; Cardim, N.; Delgado, V.; Di Salvo, G.; Donal, E.; Sade, L.E.; Ernande, L.; Garbi, M.; et al. Standardization of adult transthoracic echocardiography reporting in agreement with recent chamber quantification, diastolic function, and heart valve disease recommendations: An expert consensus document of the European Association of Cardiovascular Imaging. *Eur. Heart J. Cardiovasc. Imaging* **2017**, *18*, 1301–1310. [PubMed]
17. Roemer, S.; Jaglan, A.; Santos, D.; Umland, M.; Jain, R.; Tajik, A.J.; Khandheria, B.K. The Utility of Myocardial Work in Clinical Practice. *J. Am. Soc. Echocardiogr.* **2021**, *34*, 807–818. [CrossRef]
18. Chan, J.; Edwards, N.F.A.; Scalia, G.M.; Khandheria, B.K. Myocardial Work: A New Type of Strain Imaging? *J. Am. Soc. Echocardiogr.* **2020**, *33*, 1209–1211. [CrossRef]
19. Charfeddine, S.; Abid, L.; Hammami, R.; Bahloul, A.; Triki, F.; Kammoun, S. Left ventricular myocardial function in hemodialysis patients: The effects of preload decrease in conventional, Doppler and speckle tracking echocardiography parameters. *Pan Afr. Med. J.* **2021**, *38*, 45. [CrossRef]
20. Manganaro, R.; Marchetta, S.; Dulgheru, R.; Ilardi, F.; Sugimoto, T.; Robinet, S.; Cimino, S.; Go, Y.Y.; Bernard, A.; Kacharava, G.; et al. Echocardiographic reference ranges for normal non-invasive myocardial work indices: Results from the EACVI NORRE study. *Eur. Heart J. Cardiovasc. Imaging* **2019**, *20*, 582–590. [CrossRef]
21. Nyberg, J.; Jakobsen, E.O.; Østvik, A.; Holte, E.; Stølen, S.; Lovstakken, L.; Grenne, B.; Dalen, H. Echocardiographic Reference Ranges of Global Longitudinal Strain for All Cardiac Chambers Using Guideline-Directed Dedicated Views. *Cardiovasc. Imaging* **2023**, *16*, 1516–1531. [CrossRef]
22. Kou, S.; Caballero, L.; Dulgheru, R.; Voilliot, D.; De Sousa, C.; Kacharava, G.; Athanassopoulos, G.D.; Barone, D.; Baroni, M.; Cardim, N.; et al. Echocardiographic reference ranges for normal cardiac chamber size: Results from the NORRE study. *Eur. Heart J. Cardiovasc. Imaging* **2014**, *15*, 680–690. [CrossRef]
23. Dutta, T.; Aronow, W.S. Echocardiographic evaluation of the right ventricle: Clinical implications. *Clin. Cardiol.* **2017**, *40*, 542–548. [CrossRef] [PubMed]
24. Tamborini, G.; Marsan, N.A.; Gripari, P.; Maffessanti, F.; Brusoni, D.; Muratori, M.; Caiani, E.G.; Fiorentini, C.; Pepi, M. Reference values for right ventricular volumes and ejection fraction with real-time three-dimensional echocardiography: Evaluation in a large series of normal subjects. *J. Am. Soc. Echocardiogr.* **2010**, *23*, 109–115. [CrossRef] [PubMed]
25. Sugimoto, T.; Dulgheru, R.; Bernard, A.; Ilardi, F.; Contu, L.; Addetia, K.; Caballero, L.; Akhaladze, N.; Athanassopoulos, G.D., Barone, D.; et al. Echocardiographic reference ranges for normal left ventricular 2D strain: Results from the EACVI NORRE study. *Eur. Heart J. Cardiovasc. Imaging* **2017**, *18*, 833–840. [CrossRef] [PubMed]
26. Mostovaya, I.M.; Bots, M.L.; van den Dorpel, M.A.; Grooteman, M.P.; Kamp, O.; Levesque, R.; Ter Wee, P.M.; Nubé, M.J.; Blankestijn, P.J. A randomized trial of hemodiafiltration and change in cardiovascular parameters. *Clin. J. Am. Soc. Nephrol.* **2014**, *9*, 520–526. [CrossRef] [PubMed]
27. Czifra, A.; Páll, A.; Kulcsár, J.; Barta, K.; Kertész, A.; Paragh, G.; Lőrincz, I.; Jenei, Z.; Agarwal, A.; Zarjou, A.; et al. Hemodialysis and hemodiafiltration differently modulate left ventricular diastolic function. *BMC Nephrol.* **2013**, *14*, 76. [CrossRef] [PubMed]
28. Ethier, I.; Auger, D.; Beaulieu, M.; Wesolowska, E.; Lévesque, R. Evolution of high-sensitivity troponin-T and echocardiography parameters in patients undergoing high efficiency on-line hemodiafiltration versus conventional low-flux hemodialysis. *PLoS ONE* **2019**, *14*, e0223957. [CrossRef]
29. Hameed, I.; Gaudino, M.; Naik, A.; Rahouma, M.; Robinson, N.B.; Ruan, Y.; Demetres, M.; Bossola, M. Comparison of the effects of hemodialysis and hemodiafiltration on left ventricular hypertrophy in end-stage renal disease patients: A systematic review and meta-analysis. *Semin. Dial.* **2020**, *33*, 120–126. [CrossRef]
30. Ravera, M.; Rosa, G.M.; Fontanive, P.; Bussalino, E.; Dorighi, U.; Picciotto, D.; Di Lullo, L.; Dini, F.L.; Paoletti, E. Impaired Left Ventricular Global Longitudinal Strain among Patients with Chronic Kidney Disease and End-Stage Renal Disease and Renal Transplant Recipients. *Cardiorenal Med.* **2018**, *9*, 61–68. [CrossRef]
31. Sun, M.; Kang, Y.; Cheng, L.; Pan, C.; Cao, X.; Yao, H.; Dong, L.; Shu, X. Global longitudinal strain is an independent predictor of cardiovascular events in patients with maintenance hemodialysis: A prospective study using three-dimensional speckle tracking echocardiography. *Int. J. Cardiovasc. Imaging* **2016**, *32*, 757–766. [CrossRef] [PubMed]

32. Tamulėnaitė, E.; Žvirblytė, R.; Ereminienė, R.; Žiginskienė, E.; Ereminienė, E. Changes of Left and Right Ventricle Mechanics and Function in Patients with End-Stage Renal Disease Undergoing Haemodialysis. *Medicina* **2018**, *54*, 87. [CrossRef] [PubMed]
33. Huang, S.-H.S.; Crowley, L.E.; Jefferies, H.J.; Eldehni, M.T.; Odudu, A.; McIntyre, C.W. The Impact of Hemodialysis on Segmental and Global Longitudinal Myocardial Strain. *Can. J. Cardiol.* **2014**, *30*, 1422–1428. [CrossRef] [PubMed]
34. Kikuchi, K.; Hamano, T.; Wada, A.; Nakai, S.; Masakane, I. Predilution online hemodiafiltration is associated with improved survival compared with hemodialysis. *Kidney Int.* **2019**, *95*, 929–938. [CrossRef]
35. Takayama, F.; Miyazaki, S.; Morita, T.; Hirasawa, Y.; Niwa, T. Dialysis-related amyloidosis of the heart in long-term hemodialysis patients. *Kidney Int.* **2001**, *78*, S172–S176. [CrossRef] [PubMed]
36. Zito, C.; Longobardo, L.; Citro, R.; Alderisi, M.; Oreto, L.; Carerj, M.L.; Manganaro, R.; Cusmà-Piccione, M.; Todaro, M.C.; Di Bella, G.; et al. Ten Years of 2D Longitudinal Strain for Early Myocardial Dysfunction Detection: A Clinical Overview. *BioMed Res. Int.* **2018**, *2018*, 8979407. [CrossRef]
37. Chen, K.W.; Hsieh, W.T.; Huang, C.Y.; Huang, C.C.; Liang, H.Y.; Wang, G.J. Estimated left ventricular pressure-myocardial strain loop as an index of cardiac work predicts all-cause mortality in patients receiving regular hemodialysis. *J. Diabetes Complicat.* **2021**, *35*, 107890. [CrossRef]
38. Kamal, A.; Ahmed, N.; Zahran, A.; Ebrahim, D. Assessment of left ventricular function in patients with chronic renal failure undergoing hemodialysis. *Menoufia Med. J.* **2021**, *34*, 433.
39. Boe, E.; Skulstad, H.; Smiseth, O.A. Myocardial work by echocardiography: A novel method ready for clinical testing. *Eur. Heart J. Cardiovasc. Imaging* **2019**, *20*, 18–20. [CrossRef]
40. Guo, Y.; Tan, X.; Li, Z.; Dai, C.; Yang, Q.; Nie, Y.; Cao, X.; Shu, X.; Pan, C.; Sun, M. Global left ventricular myocardial work: A novel method to assess left ventricular myocardial function and predict major adverse cardiovascular events in maintenance hemodialysis patients. *J. Clin. Ultrasound* **2024**, 1–10. [CrossRef]
41. Paneni, F.; Gregori, M.; Ciavarella, G.M.; Sciarretta, S.; De Biase, L.; Marino, L.; Tocci, G.; Principe, F.; Domenici, A.; Luciani, R.; et al. Right ventricular dysfunction in patients with end-stage renal disease. *Am. J. Nephrol.* **2010**, *32*, 432–438. [CrossRef] [PubMed]
42. Zoccali, C.; Benedetto, F.A.; Mallamaci, F.; Ripepi, G.; Giacone, G.; Cataliotti, A.; Seminara, G.; Stancanelli, B.; Malatino, L.S. Prognostic impact of the indexation of left ventricular mass in patients undergoing dialysis. *J. Am. Soc. Nephrol.* **2001**, *12*, 2768–2774. [CrossRef] [PubMed]
43. Mostovaya, I.M.; Bots, M.L.; van den Dorpel, M.A.; Goldschmeding, R.; den Hoedt, C.H.; Kamp, O.; Levesque, R.; Mazairac, A.H.; Penne, E.L.; Swinkels, D.W.; et al. Left Ventricular Mass in Dialysis Patients, Determinants and Relation with Outcome. Results from the COnvective TRansport STudy (CONTRAST). *PLoS ONE* **2014**, *9*, e84587. [CrossRef] [PubMed]
44. Francisco, R.C.; Aloha, M.; Ramón, P.S. Effects of high-efficiency postdilution online hemodiafiltration and high-flux hemodialysis on serum phosphorus and cardiac structure and function in patients with end-stage renal disease. *Int. Urol. Nephrol.* **2013**, *45*, 1373–1378. [CrossRef]
45. Schiffl, H.; Lang, S.M.; Fischer, R. Effects of high efficiency post-dilution on-line hemodiafiltration or conventional hemodialysis on residual renal function and left ventricular hypertrophy. *Int. Urol. Nephrol.* **2013**, *45*, 1389–1396. [CrossRef]

medicina

MDPI

Article

Bleeding and Thrombotic Events in Hemodialysis Patients with Atrial Fibrillation on Anticoagulation and Antiplatelet Therapy: A 24-Month Cohort Study

Zorica M. Dimitrijevic [1,2,*], Branka P. Mitic [1,2], Danijela D. Tasic [1], Tamara Vrecic [1], Karolina Paunovic [1,2] and Sonja Salinger [2,3]

[1] Clinic for Nephrology, University Clinical Center Nis, 18000 Nis, Serbia
[2] Medical Faculty, University of Nis, 18000 Nis, Serbia
[3] Clinic for Cardiovascular Disesase, Univeristy Clinical Center Nis, 18000 Nis, Serbia
* Correspondence: zorica_mdimitrijevic@yahoo.com; Tel.: +381-638335284

Abstract: *Background and Objectives*: Patients undergoing chronic hemodialysis (HD) are predisposed to both thrombotic and bleeding complications due to the complex interplay of end-stage renal disease (ESRD), cardiovascular comorbidities, and the routine use of anticoagulant and antiplatelet therapies. This study aimed to investigate the incidence of bleeding and thrombotic events in chronic HD patients receiving anticoagulant and antiplatelet therapy, with a specific focus on those with atrial fibrillation (AF). *Materials and Methods*: A total of 224 patients, with 43 (19%) of them diagnosed with AF, were included in this single-center, observational cohort study conducted over 24 months. The cohort was divided into three groups: patients without anticoagulation, those on warfarin monotherapy, and those on combined warfarin and aspirin therapy. Bleeding events were classified as major, clinically relevant non-major bleeding (CRNMB), or minor bleeding, while thrombotic events included ischemic stroke, myocardial infarction, pulmonary embolism, and arteriovenous fistula thrombosis. *Results*: Overall, 35.7% of patients experienced a bleeding event, with major bleeding occurring in 9.4%. Patients with AF had significantly higher rates of major bleeding (18.6%) compared to those without AF (7.18%; $p = 0.043$), especially in the combined therapy group. Mortality due to bleeding was also higher in AF patients (14%). In contrast, thrombotic events occurred in 26.8% of patients, with AF patients experiencing significantly more events (48.8%) compared to non-AF patients (21.5%; $p = 0.0006$). The hazard ratio (HR) for major bleeding in patients on combined warfarin and aspirin therapy was 2.56 ($p = 0.016$), while the HR for thrombotic events was 2.34 ($p = 0.0202$). *Conclusions*: These findings highlight the increased risks of both bleeding and thrombosis in chronic HD patients with AF, particularly those on combined anticoagulation and antiplatelet therapy.

Keywords: hemodialysis; atrial fibrillation; anticoagulation therapy; bleeding; thrombosis

1. Introduction

End-stage kidney disease (ESKD) is a serious condition that necessitates continuous therapy with permanent hemodialysis (HD) procedures. While HD is a life-saving treatment, it is accompanied by various complications, especially those related to bleeding and thrombosis. These complications arise due to the complex interaction of cardiovascular comorbidities, the uremic environment, and the use of anticoagulant and antiplatelet therapy. While anticoagulation is mainly used to prevent thrombosis, it significantly increases the risk of bleeding. This bleeding tendency in patients with ESKD is multifactorial and associated with the reduced clearance of anticoagulants in patients with impaired renal function, leading to increased drug levels [1], uremic platelet dysfunction [2,3], impaired platelet–vessel wall interactions, renal anemia, and the chronic use of heparin during dialysis sessions. Establishing a balance between preventing thrombosis and mitigating the risk of bleeding represents a significant clinical challenge in treating these patients [4].

Atrial fibrillation (AF), one of the most common cardiovascular comorbidities in patients with ESKD, occurs in 3.8–27% of chronic HD patients, with the prevalence varying with age, cardiovascular health, and comorbid conditions such as hypertension and diabetes [5,6]. As AF increases the risk of thromboembolism, oral anticoagulation for stroke prevention is indicated in the vast majority of ESKD patients with AF. However, the studies on the benefit of anticoagulation in dialysis patients are inconclusive, and an excessive risk of bleeding during vitamin K antagonist treatment is observed [7–9]. Additionally, in some cases, antiplatelet agents are added to the treatment regimen, especially for those with ischemic heart disease. However, the combined use of anticoagulants and antiplatelet agents is associated with a further exacerbated risk of bleeding, including life-threatening episodes of intracranial and gastrointestinal bleeding [10].

As a result, clinicians encounter challenging therapeutic dilemmas in balancing the risk of thromboembolism and bleeding. The dual risks associated with anticoagulation therapy in HD patients with AF have been well documented. For example, while anticoagulant therapy is effective in reducing the incidence of cerebrovascular accidents and ischemic strokes, it can also lead to severe hemorrhagic complications, especially in patients on combination therapy [11]. This dilemma is further exacerbated by the advanced age and comorbidities of HD patients, who are often more susceptible to thrombotic and bleeding complications. Despite these risks, the optimal approach to anticoagulant treatment in this population remains unclear, with different guidelines and practices depending on the local protocols and patient characteristics. Previous studies have documented the effectiveness of anticoagulant therapy in reducing ischemic events, but this benefit is often balanced by an increased incidence of hemorrhagic complications, especially in patients receiving combination therapy [12]. Given these challenges, the optimal strategy for anticoagulation management in HD patients with AF remains a subject of ongoing debate, with variations in treatment protocols based on patient characteristics, local guidelines, and clinical judgment.

This study aimed to further investigate the incidence of bleeding and thrombosis in chronic HD patients receiving anticoagulant and antiplatelet therapy, with a particular focus on those diagnosed with AF.

2. Materials and Methods

This single-center, observational cohort study was conducted over a 24-month period and approved by the Ethics Committee of Nis University Hospital (approval number 39454; 1 November 2019). The study adhered to the principles outlined in the Declaration of Helsinki. All the participants provided informed consent, both oral and written, prior to their inclusion in the study.

The data on concomitant diseases and pharmacological treatments were extracted from electronic medical records, including hospital admissions, outpatient visits, and complete laboratory tests. The study team systematically reviewed the patients' medical documentation, including discharge letters, each month to monitor for bleeding or thrombotic events.

2.1. Outcomes and Definitions

The primary outcome of the study was the incidence of new bleeding events.

Major bleeding was defined as by the International Society on Thrombosis and Haemostasis (ISTH), i.e., fatal bleeding and/or symptomatical bleeding in a critical area or organ, such as intracranial, intraspinal, intraocular, retroperitoneal, intraarticular, or pericardial, or intramuscular with compartment syndrome, or a drop in hemoglobin of at least 20 g/L for the last 24 h period, and/or bleeding or leading to transfusion of two or more units of whole blood or red blood cells [13].

Clinically relevant non-major bleeding (CRNMB) was defined as bleeding that did not fulfill the major bleed criteria but led to hospitalization, any intervention (medical or surgical), unscheduled visit, or change in antithrombotic therapy [14].

Minor bleeding was defined as non-life-threatening bleeding events that did not necessitate medical intervention.

Secondary outcomes included arterial and venous thrombosis events, categorized into ischemic stroke (IS), myocardial infarction (MI), pulmonary thromboembolism (PTE), and arteriovenous fistula (AVF) thrombosis. Thrombotic events (IS, MI, and PTE) were diagnosed using a combination of clinical presentation, imaging modalities (such as CT or ultrasound), and laboratory biomarkers (e.g., troponins, D-dimers) based on the standard hospital protocols for each condition. AVF thrombosis was diagnosed through clinical examination (e.g., absence of bruit or thrill) and confirmed by using Doppler ultrasound imaging.

Mortality data, including death attributable to bleeding or thrombotic events, were collected throughout the 24-month follow-up period.

2.2. Study Population

Patients were recruited among incident HD patients and were selected based on the predefined inclusion and exclusion criteria. All the patients receiving chronic HD at our center were eligible for inclusion if they were 18 years or older, had been on HD for at least three months, and were able to provide informed consent. The exclusion criteria included patients with active cancer, known coagulation disorders unrelated to renal disease, or contraindications to anticoagulation therapy and patients with recent surgery or critical illnesses. Of the initial 254 patients screened, 224 met the inclusion criteria after excluding those with contraindications (Figure 1).

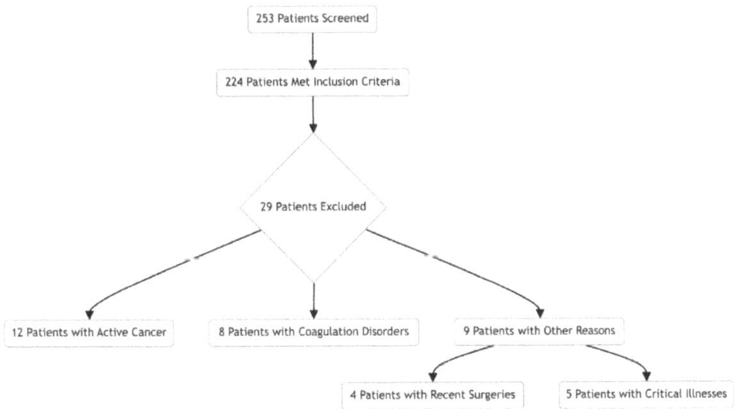

Figure 1. Flowchart diagram of the study cohort creation.

2.3. Sample Size and Power Analysis

A power analysis was conducted prior to the study to determine the minimum sample size required to detect the meaningful differences in bleeding and thrombotic events between patients with atrial fibrillation (AF) and those without. Based on prior studies and the anticipated event rates of bleeding and thrombosis in HD patients, an estimated sample size of 200 patients would provide 80% power to detect a hazard ratio of 2.0 with a two-sided alpha of 0.05. With 224 patients included in the study, of whom 19% had AF, the study was adequately powered to detect the clinically significant differences in bleeding and thrombotic outcomes between the groups.

2.4. Anticoagulation and Antiplatelet Therapy

The patients were divided into three groups based on their anticoagulant and antiplatelet treatment regimen:

Group 1: Patients not receiving any anticoagulant or antiplatelet agents.

Group 2: Patients on warfarin monotherapy.

Group 3: Patients receiving both warfarin and aspirin for anticoagulation and antiplatelet therapy, respectively.

The treating physician guided the choice of therapy, considering each patient's cardiovascular risk profile, comorbidities, and AF status.

Warfarin doses were adjusted based on monthly INR testing, with the goal of maintaining a therapeutic range of 2.0–3.0. All the patients underwent INR testing once a month, and dosages were modified accordingly to ensure effective anticoagulation while minimizing the risk of bleeding or thrombotic events. Although factors such as body weight and renal function were not explicitly used for dose adjustments, the INR monitoring provided a reliable measure to capture any changes related to these factors, allowing for appropriate dose modifications when necessary.

Aspirin was administered at a standard daily dose of 75–100 mg.

2.5. Statistical Analysis

Continuous variables were expressed as mean $\pm$ standard deviation (SD) or median with interquartile range (IQR), depending on the data distribution. Categorical variables were summarized as frequencies and percentages. The differences between the groups were analyzed using the chi-square test for categorical variables and the independent t-test or Mann–Whitney U test for continuous variables, as appropriate. Kaplan–Meier survival curves were generated to estimate the cumulative incidence of bleeding and thrombotic events over the 24-month follow-up. Cox proportional hazard models were used to identify the independent predictors of bleeding and thrombosis, adjusting for potential confounders such as age, gender, comorbidities, and treatment type. The assumption of proportional hazards for the Cox models was verified using Schoenfeld residuals. The global and individual tests for covariates showed no significant violations of the proportional hazards assumption ($p > 0.05$ for all tests). Log-minus-log survival plots were visually inspected, and no deviations from proportionality were observed. Therefore, the Cox proportional hazards model was considered appropriate for identifying the predictors of bleeding and thrombotic events in this cohort.

Statistical significance was set at $p < 0.05$, and all the analyses were performed using SPSS statistical software (version 26.0, IBM Corp., Armonk, NY, USA).

3. Results

A total of 224 patients undergoing chronic HD were included in the study. The median age of the cohort was 61 years (IQR 19–89), with 63.8% of the patients being male. The median duration of dialysis was 66.3 months (range: 7–299 months). Among the study population, 19% had atrial fibrillation (AF). The patients with AF were significantly older (median age of 64.7 years vs. 58 years for those without AF, $p = 0.038$) and had a higher prevalence of previous cardiovascular incidents, such as ischemic stroke (23.3% vs. 5%, $p = 0.002$). Among the patients with AF, 24 (55.8%) were treated with warfarin monotherapy, while 19 (44.2%) were on a combination of warfarin and aspirin therapy. Table 1 summarizes the baseline characteristics of the study population.

Table 1. Baseline characteristics of the study population.

	All Patients	Without AF	With AF			
			Total	Warfarin + Aspirin	Warfarin	*p*-Value
Total number of patients	224	181	43 (19%)	19 (44.2%)	24 (55.8%)	
Men (%)	143 (63.8%)	100 (55.2%)	30 (69.7%)	9 (20.9%)	21 (48.4)	0.036
Age, median (IQR)	61 (19–89.0)	58.0 (19–77)	64.7 (46–89.0)	70.0 (51.0–89.0)	68.3 (43.5–76.0)	0.038
Duration of dialysis, months	66.3 (5–299)	46.3(5–173)	60.3 (89–221.0)	42.6 (25.6–202)	58.3 (31.7–198.0)	0.036
Comorbidities, *n* (%)						
Previous CVI	20 (8.9%)	10 (5%)	10 (23.3%)	2 (4.6%)	8 (18.6%)	0.002
Ischemic heart disease	33 (12.4%)	19 (10.%)	14 (32%)	6 (13.9%)	8 (18.6%)	0.71
HTA (Hypertension)	185 (69.3%)	173 (95.5%)	12 (27.9%)	5 (11.6%)	7 (16.2%)	0.75
Heart failure	43(19.9%)	37 (20.4%)	7 (16.2%)	4 (9.3%)	3 (6.9%)	0.36
Diabetes	68 (30.3%)	35 (51.4%)	33 (48.55)	20 (60.6%)	13 (39.4%)	0.022
Blood chemistry						
Hemoglobin g/L	103.2 + 11.5	102.1 ± 11.4	103.2 ± 11.1	101.3 + 10.1	102.1 + 10.2	0.9
White blood cells count, $\times 10^9$/L	6.2 + 2.4	6.1 ± 2.1	6.3 ± 1.7	7.1 + 2.5	6.4 + 1.1	0.9
Platelet count, $\times 10^9$/L	164.3 + 68.2	197.1 ± 50.2	170.5 ± 41.1	146.4 + 61.4	131.0 + 40.9	0.63
INR (PT)	1.6 + 0.4	1.3 ± 0.2	1.5.0 ± 0.1	2.0 + 0.4	2.4 + 0.1	0.09
aPTT (seconds)	33.6 + 13.7	32.2 ± 11.3	31.8 ± 13.1	33.3 + 4.6	38.8 + 9.4	0.68
Fibrinogen (g/L)	5.0 + 1.2	4.2 ± 1.2	5.2 ± 1.4	5.6 + 1.4	5.4 + 1.2	0.88
Medications						
RAAS blockers	135 (74.5%)	100 (55.2%)	35 (81.3%)	10 (23.3%)	24 (55.8%)	0.07
Calcium blockers	106 (58.5%)	84 (46.4%)	22 (51.1%)	10 (23.3%)	12 (27.9%)	0.06
Statins	31 (17.1%)	15 (8.2%)	16 (37.2%)	8 (18.6%)	8 (18.6%)	0.61

Abbreviations: AF—atrial fibrillation; CVI—cerebrovascular insult; RAAS—renin-angiotensin-aldosterone.

3.1. Bleeding Events

During the follow-up period, a total of 80 patients (35.7%) experienced at least one bleeding event. Among these, 21 patients (9.4%) had major bleeding episodes, 23 patients (10.3%) had clinically relevant non-major bleeding, while 24 patients (10.7%) had minor bleeding. Twelve patients (5.3%) died due to bleeding-related complications. The data are presented in Table 2.

In the AF subgroup, bleeding events occurred in 22 patients (51.2%). The patients with AF had a notably higher percentage of any bleeding compared to those without AF, and the difference was statistically significant ($p = 0.029$). The odds ratio (OR) for any bleeding event in the patients with AF compared to those without AF was 2.21 (95% CI: 1.10–4.43), indicating that the AF patients were more than twice as likely to experience a bleeding event. Major bleeding occurred in 8 patients (18.6%) with AF and in 13 patients (7.18%) without AF ($p = 0.043$), with an OR of 2.92 (95% CI: 1.15–7.44), suggesting an almost threefold increased risk of major bleeding in the patients with AF.

Table 2. Bleeding events by patient subgroup.

Bleeding Outcome	All the Patients (n = 224)	Without AF (n = 181)	With AF (n = 43)	p Value
Any bleeding	80 (35.7%)	58 (32.4%)	22(51.2%)	0.029
• Major bleeding	21 (9.4%)	13 (7.18%)	8 (18.6%)	0.043
• Clinically relevant bleeding	23 (10.3%)	20 (11.4%)	3 (7.0%)	0.61
• Minor bleeding	24 (10.7%)	19 (10.5%)	5 (11.6%)	1
Death due to bleeding	12 (5.3%)	6 (3.3%)	6 (14%)	0.016

During the follow-up period, major bleeding occurred more frequently in the patients on combined warfarin and aspirin therapy compared to those on warfarin monotherapy. Specifically, 18.6% of the patients on combined therapy experienced major bleeding, compared to 7.18% of the patients on warfarin alone (p = 0.016). The OR for major bleeding in the patients receiving combined warfarin and aspirin therapy was 2.56 (95% CI: 1.43–4.66), indicating a more than twofold increased risk of major bleeding in this group compared to that on warfarin monotherapy. For CRNMB, the OR for the patients on combined therapy was 2.34 (95% CI: 1.46–6.13, p = 0.0202), compared to those on warfarin alone. These results suggest that combination therapy significantly elevates the risk of both major and non-major bleeding.

A total of 12 patients (5.3%) died due to bleeding-related complications during the study period. Among those, seven patients (14%) were in the warfarin group, and five patients (3.3%) were in the non-warfarin group. The odds ratio (OR) for bleeding-related death in the warfarin group compared to the non-warfarin group was 4.72 (95% CI: 1.38–16.16, p = 0.016). The higher rate of fatal outcomes in the AF patients underscores the heightened bleeding risk in this subgroup, particularly among those receiving aggressive anticoagulation therapy.

3.2. Thrombotic Events

A total of 60 thrombotic events in 42 patients occurred during the study period, representing 26.8% of the cohort. In contrast to the increased risk of bleeding, the AF patients also faced a markedly higher risk of thrombotic events, with nearly half of the patients with AF (48.8%) experiencing at least one thrombotic event compared to 21.5% of the non-AF patients. Ischemic stroke and myocardial infarction were the most common thrombotic events, with the AF patients being significantly more likely to suffer from these complications. The rate of ischemic stroke in the AF patients (18.6%) was much higher than in those without AF (3.86%, p = 0.0117), reflecting the well-established link between AF and thromboembolism. Similarly, MI occurred in 11.6% of the AF patients compared to 2.8% of the non-AF patients (Table 3).

Thrombotic events contributed to a significant number of deaths in the study population. Overall, 12 patients (5.35%) died due to thrombosis-related complications. Similar to the findings for major bleeding, the patients with AF had a much higher mortality rate from thrombotic events (16.2%) compared to those without AF (2.8%, p = 0.0016). The higher mortality in the AF patients suggests that thrombosis is a leading cause of death in this subgroup, despite the use of anticoagulation therapy.

Table 3. Thrombotic events by patient subgroup.

Thrombotic Outcome	All the Patients (n = 224)	Without AF (n = 181)	With AF (n = 43)	p Value
Any thrombotic event	60 (26.8%)	39 (21.5%)	21 (48.8%)	0.0006
• Ischemic stroke	15 (6.7%)	7 (3.86%)	8(18.6%)	0.0117
• AVF thrombosis	28 (12.5%)	21 (11.6%)	7(16.2%)	0.563
• Myocardial infarction	10 (4.5%)	5 (2.8%)	5 (11.6%)	0.034
• PTE	7 (3.5)	6(3.3)	1 (2.32)	1
Death due to thrombosis	12 (5.35%)	5 (2.8%)	7 (16.2%)	0.0016

Abbreviations: AVF—arteriovenous fistula; PTE—pulmonary thromboembolism.

3.3. Overall Mortality

The mortality due to all causes was significantly higher in the patients with AF, with 14% of the deaths attributable to bleeding and 16.2% to thrombotic events. The hazard ratios (HR) for major bleeding and thrombotic events in the patients on combined warfarin and aspirin therapy were elevated, with an HR of 2.56 for major bleeding (p = 0.016) and 2.34 for clinically relevant bleeding (p = 0.0202) (Table 4). Warfarin monotherapy, while still associated with major bleeding, was not as strongly predictive of such events compared to the combined therapy. The patients on warfarin monotherapy had a lower incidence of thrombotic events than those on the combined therapy but still faced a notable risk of ischemic stroke (HR = 0.81, p = 0.11). The combined therapy group had a significantly higher rate of thrombotic events compared to the other two groups. This group had elevated hazard ratios for thrombotic events, including myocardial infarction (HR = 0.76, p = 0.1) and ischemic stroke (HR = 0.72, p = 0.683), although statistical significance was not reached in all the cases. The trend suggests that while the combined therapy may reduce some thrombotic risks, it does not fully mitigate them, and the increased risk of bleeding must also be considered.

Table 4. Hazard ratios for thrombotic and bleeding events in the patients on warfarin and the combined warfarin–aspirin therapy.

	Warfarin		Warfarin + Aspirin	
	HR (95% CI)	p-Value	HR (95% CI)	p-Value
Thrombotic event				
• Myocardial infarction	081 (0.52–0.89)	0.11	0.76 (0.67–1.28)	0.1
• PTE	0.86 (0.75–1.45)	0.361	0.88 (0.62–1.13)	0.378
• Ischemic stroke	0.77 (0.41–1.67)	0.479	0.72 (0.05–1.63)	0.683
Bleeding				
• Major bleeding	1.14 (0.92–3.12)	0.684	2.56 (1.43–4.66)	0.016
• Clinically relevant bleeding	1.31(1.11–2.81)	0.254	2.34 (1.46–6.13)	0.0202
• Minor bleeding	0.91 (0.76–1.60)	0.62	1.01 (0.91–1.28)	0.90
All cause deaths	1.79 (1.45–3.7)	0.0148	1.98 (1.68–5.12)	0.0163

Abbreviations: PTE—pulmonary thromboembolism.

4. Discussion

The findings of this study highlight a significantly enhanced risk of both bleeding and thrombotic events in chronic HD patients with AF, especially those on combined warfarin and aspirin therapy. The risk of major bleeding in the AF patients (18.6%) was notably higher compared to the non-AF patients (7.18%, p = 0.043), a result consistent with the current literature. Two independent studies similarly reported a significantly elevated risk of bleeding complications in dialysis patients receiving anticoagulation therapy, particularly among those treated with combined anticoagulants [15,16].

In the present study, the risk of major bleeding was more pronounced in the patients on the combined warfarin and aspirin therapy (18.6%) than in those receiving the warfarin monotherapy (7.18%, $p = 0.016$). The combined warfarin and aspirin therapy, while beneficial in reducing thrombotic risk, significantly increased the hazard ratio (HR = 2.56, $p = 0.016$) for major bleeding events compared to the warfarin monotherapy (HR = 1.14, $p = 0.684$). This finding is consistent with the results from a systematic review by Lei et al., which demonstrated that warfarin significantly increases the risks of major bleeding, including hemorrhagic stroke, in hemodialysis patients [12]. Comparable trends have been observed in other studies where the authors reported that combined anticoagulant and antiplatelet therapy was associated with a higher risk of major bleeding events in patients with chronic kidney disease (CKD), which aligns with the findings of this study [17,18]. Additionally, Daimon et al. found that bleeding risks were significantly elevated in hemodialysis patients using warfarin and aspirin, with a bleeding event rate of 9.81 per 10,000 patient-days for warfarin and 7.37 for aspirin [19].

The increased risk of thrombotic events in AF patients, particularly ischemic stroke and myocardial infarction, was another key finding of our study. Nearly half of the AF patients (48.8%) experienced a thrombotic event; 18.6% of them suffered from ischemic stroke compared to 3.86% in the non-AF patients.

This is concordant with the well-established association between AF and thromboembolic events in HD patients. Olesen et al. also found a marked increase in ischemic stroke risk in HD patients with AF, stressing the vulnerability of this patient population [20]. Our results further emphasize the potential dangers when aspirin is added to the treatment regimen.

On the other hand, the rate of myocardial infarction was remarkably higher in the AF patients (11.6%) compared to those without AF (2.8%, $p = 0.034$). Earlier research supports this finding, noting that AF is a potent risk factor for cardiovascular events, including MI, in CKD and dialysis patients [21].

Overall, the thrombotic event-related mortality among the AF patients (16.2%) was alarmingly high, echoing the results of the recent research reporting correspondingly high mortality rates associated with thrombotic complications in this population [22].

In contrast to other reports that suggested that warfarin monotherapy could effectively reduce the thrombotic risk without a disproportionate increase in bleeding [23,24], our findings indicate that warfarin monotherapy still carries a substantial bleeding risk. However, the bleeding risk was comparatively lower than with combined therapy.

Interestingly, despite the elevated risk of thrombotic events in the patients on combined warfarin and aspirin therapy, the risk reduction was not statistically significant in some cases, suggesting that while combined therapy may pose reduced thrombotic risks, it exposes one to significant bleeding risks. This finding is consistent with the results from prior studies which reported similar trends in anticoagulated CKD populations [25,26].

Our findings significantly impact the anticoagulation management in HD patients, especially those with AF. The study shows that although anticoagulant therapy, particularly warfarin in combination with aspirin, may provide some protection against thrombotic events, it is also associated with a high rate of bleeding complications, including major bleeding and bleeding-related mortality. This is remarkably relevant for patients with a history of cerebrovascular incidents, who showed an even higher bleeding risk when treated with the combined therapy. The increased risk of these events in this population reaffirms the need for meticulous patient evaluation and individualization of antithrombotic therapy.

Given these findings, clinicians need to carefully assess the risk–benefit ratio for anticoagulation among HD patients. Current recommendations for AF anticoagulation may underestimate the potential bleeding risk in HD patients, highlighting the need for more tailored guidelines. For instance, a critical area for future research is the development of more refined risk stratification tools to identify HD patients who are most likely to benefit from anticoagulation while minimizing the adverse outcomes. The current risk models, such as the CHA_2DS_2-VASc and HAS-BLED scores, may not fully capture the unique bleeding and thrombotic risks in patients with ESKD, highlighting the need for tailored scoring systems that better reflect the clinical complexness of this population. Given these risks, recent studies have highlighted the potential alternatives to warfarin, such as Direct Oral Anticoagulants (DOACs), which may provide a safer profile for patients with CKD. For example, the IRIS registry demonstrated the efficacy of rivaroxaban in reducing thromboembolic risk with potentially fewer bleeding complications in patients with CKD [27]. Additionally, the REGUEIFA registry, a multicenter study comparing vitamin K antagonists (such as warfarin) with DOACs, found that patients on DOACs reported higher satisfaction and a better health-related quality of life, as well as a lower incidence of adverse events, particularly bleeding [28].

A recent systematic review and meta-analysis conducted by de Lucena et al. [29], compared the efficacy and safety of DOACs with vitamin K antagonists in patients with AF on chronic hemodialysis. Their findings indicated that DOACs, particularly apixaban, were associated with a reduced risk of major bleeding compared to warfarin, without a significant increase in thromboembolic events. The study also suggested that DOACs offer a favorable safety profile in this high-risk population despite the concerns about their use in patients with advanced CKD due to the altered pharmacokinetics.

These findings support the growing body of literature suggesting that DOACs could be a viable alternative to warfarin in patients with CKD and AF, particularly those at high risk of bleeding. However, the use of DOACs in ESKD remains somewhat controversial, as not all DOACs have been extensively studied in this population.

Further research is needed to solidify the role of DOACs in this population, but the current evidence suggests that they may help balance the prevention of thrombotic events with the reduction in bleeding risk, a major challenge in managing AF in CKD patients.

Finally, further research is needed to explore the impact of combination therapy with anticoagulants and antiplatelet agents. Although our findings suggest an increased bleeding risk in patients on warfarin and aspirin, it is unclear whether this combination provides sufficient thrombotic protection to justify the higher risk of bleeding. Prospective studies comparing different anticoagulation strategies, including monotherapy versus combination therapy, are essential to guide more effective clinical decision making in this vulnerable group.

Study Limitations

There were some limitations to our study that should be acknowledged. First, this was a single-center study, and the results may not be generalizable to all HD populations. Additionally, while we were able to identify the associations between anticoagulation therapy and bleeding/thrombotic outcomes, the observational design of the study precludes the ability to infer causality. Randomized controlled trials are needed to further elucidate the optimal approach to anticoagulation in HD patients with AF and to determine whether alternative therapies, such as DOACs or individualized dosing regimens, could reduce the risk of bleeding while maintaining the thromboembolic protection.

5. Conclusions

This study reinforces the complex relationship between anticoagulation, bleeding, and thrombosis in HD patients with AF. As previously shown, patients receiving combined warfarin and aspirin therapy encounter a significantly higher risk of bleeding, while warfarin monotherapy, though less risky, still carries substantial bleeding and thrombotic risks. Clinicians must weigh these risks carefully when considering the therapeutic strategies for HD patients, especially those with AF. Future research should focus on identifying the subgroups of patients that benefit most from anticoagulant and antiplatelet therapy while minimizing the adverse outcomes, as well as exploring alternative anticoagulation strategies that offer a more favorable risk profile in this high-risk population.

Author Contributions: Conceptualization, Z.M.D. and S.S.; methodology, Z.M.D. and T.V.; software, D.D.T.; validation, K.P. and B.P.M.; formal analysis, Z.M.D. and T.V.; investigation, Z.M.D. and K.P.; resources, D.D.T.; data curation, B.P.M.; writing—original draft preparation, Z.M.D.; writing—review and editing, S.S.; visualization, T.V.; supervision, S.S.; project administration, Z.M.D. All authors have read and agreed to the published version of the manuscript.

Funding: The Study was performed under the INT-MF61 project from The Medical Faculty, University of Nis, Serbia. However, no financial grant or funding were received.

Institutional Review Board Statement: The study was conducted in accordance with the Declaration of Helsinki, and approved by the Ethics Committee of University Clinical Center Nis (approval number 39454; 1 November 2019).

Informed Consent Statement: Informed consent was obtained from all the subjects involved in the study.

Data Availability Statement: The data that support the findings of this study are available from the corresponding author upon reasonable request.

Acknowledgments: The authors would like to express their gratitude to the medical staff of the Hemodialysis Unit at the University Clinical Center Nis, Serbia, for their valuable contribution during the study.

Conflicts of Interest: The authors declare no conflicts of interest.

References

1. Catella, J.; Bertoletti, L.; Mismetti, P.; Ollier, E.; Samperiz, A.; Soler, S.; Suriñach, J.M.; Mahé, I.; Lorente, M.A.; Braester, A.; et al. Severe renal impairment and risk of bleeding during anticoagulation for venous thromboembolism. *J. Thromb. Haemost.* **2020**, *18*, 1728–1737. [CrossRef] [PubMed]
2. Escolar, G.; Díaz-Ricart, M.; Cases, A. Uremic platelet dysfunction: Past and present. *Curr. Hematol. Rep.* **2005**, *4*, 359–367. [PubMed]
3. Kozek-Langenecker, S.A.; Masaki, T.; Mohammad, H.; Green, W.; Mohammad, S.F.; Cheung, A.K. Fibrinogen fragments and platelet dysfunction in uremia. *Kidney Int.* **1999**, *56*, 299–305. [CrossRef]
4. Soler-Espejo, E.; Esteve-Pastor, M.A.; Rivera-Caravaca, J.M.; Roldan, V.; Marín, F. Reducing bleeding risk in patients on oral anticoagulation therapy. *Expert Rev. Cardiovasc. Ther.* **2023**, *21*, 923–936. [CrossRef]
5. Königsbrügge, O.; Posch, F.; Antlanger, M.; Kovarik, J.; Klauser-Braun, R.; Kletzmayr, J.; Schmaldienst, S.; Auinger, M.; Zuntner, G.; Lorenz, M.; et al. Prevalence of atrial fibrillation and antithrombotic therapy in hemodialysis patients: Cross-sectional results of the Vienna Investigation of AtriaL Fibrillation and Thromboembolism in Patients on HemoDIalysis (VIVALDI). *PLoS ONE* **2017**, *12*, e0182798.
6. Wang, E.Y.; Hulme, O.L.; Khurshid, S.; Weng, L.C.; Choi, S.H.; Walkey, A.J.; Ashburner, J.M.; McManus, D.D.; Singer, D.E.; Atlas, S.J.; et al. Initial precipitants and recurrence of atrial fibrillation. *Circ. Arrhythm. Electrophysiol.* **2020**, *13*, e007716. [CrossRef]
7. Königsbrügge, O.; Meisel, H.; Beyer, A.; Schmaldienst, S.; Klauser-Braun, R.; Lorenz, M.; Auinger, M.; Kletzmayr, J.; Hecking, M.; Winkelmayer, W.C.; et al. Anticoagulation use and the risk of stroke and major bleeding in patients on hemodialysis: From the VIVALDI, a population-based prospective cohort study. *J. Thromb. Haemost.* **2021**, *19*, 2984–2996. [CrossRef] [PubMed]
8. Van Der Meersch, H.; De Bacquer, D.; De Vriese, A.S. Vitamin K antagonists for stroke prevention in hemodialysis patients with atrial fibrillation: A systematic review and meta-analysis. *Am. Heart J.* **2017**, *184*, 37–46. [CrossRef]
9. Tan, J.; Liu, S.; Segal, J.B.; Alexander, G.C.; McAdams-DeMarco, M. Warfarin use and stroke, bleeding, and mortality risk in patients with end-stage renal disease and atrial fibrillation: A systematic review and meta-analysis. *BMC Nephrol.* **2016**, *17*, 157. [CrossRef] [PubMed]
10. Elliott, M.J.; Zimmerman, D.; Holden, R.M. Warfarin anticoagulation in hemodialysis patients: A systematic review of bleeding rates. *Am. J. Kidney Dis.* **2007**, *50*, 433–440. [CrossRef]
11. Bansal, N. Use of oral anticoagulation for patients with ESRD on hemodialysis with atrial fibrillation: Verdict 1. *Clin. J. Am. Soc. Nephrol.* **2016**, *11*, 2093–2094. [CrossRef] [PubMed] [PubMed Central]
12. Lei, H.; Yu, L.T.; Wang, W.N.; Zhang, S.G. Warfarin and the risk of death, stroke, and major bleeding in patients with atrial fibrillation receiving hemodialysis: A systematic review and meta-analysis. *Front. Pharmacol.* **2018**, *9*, 1218. [CrossRef] [PubMed]
13. Schulman, S.; Kearon, C. Definition of major bleeding in clinical investigations of antihemostatic medicinal products in non-surgical patients. *J. Thromb. Haemost.* **2005**, *3*, 692–694. [CrossRef]

14. Kaatz, S.; Ahmad, D.; Spyropoulos, A.C.; Schulman, S. Definition of clinically relevant non-major bleeding in studies of anticoagulants in atrial fibrillation and venous thromboembolic disease in non-surgical patients: Communication from the SSC of the ISTH. *J. Thromb. Haemost.* **2015**, *13*, 2119–2126. [CrossRef] [PubMed]
15. Wizemann, V.; Tong, L.; Satayathum, S.; Disney, A.; Akiba, T.; Fissell, R.B.; Kerr, P.; Young, E.W.; Robinson, B.M. Atrial fibrillation in hemodialysis patients: Clinical features and associations with anticoagulant therapy. *Kidney Int.* **2014**, *66*, 65–70. [CrossRef] [PubMed]
16. Kuno, T.; Takagi, H.; Ando, T.; Sugiyama, T.; Miyashita, S.; Valentin, N.; Shimada, Y.J.; Kodaira, M.; Numasawa, Y.; Briasoulis, A.; et al. Oral anticoagulation for patients with atrial fibrillation on long-term hemodialysis. *J. Am. Coll. Cardiol.* **2020**, *75*, 273–285. [CrossRef]
17. Chan, K.E.; Lazarus, J.M.; Thadhani, R.; Hakim, R.M. Warfarin use associates with increased risk for stroke in hemodialysis patients with atrial fibrillation. *J. Am. Soc. Nephrol.* **2015**, *20*, 2223–2233. [CrossRef]
18. Aursulesei, V.; Costache, I.I. Anticoagulation in chronic kidney disease: From guidelines to clinical practice. *Clin. Cardiol.* **2019**, *42*, 774–782. [CrossRef]
19. Daimon, S. Adverse effect of antithrombotic medications on bleeding events and comparison of antithrombotic agents in hemodialysis patients. *Ther. Apher. Dial.* **2019**, *23*, 32–37. [CrossRef]
20. Olesen, J.B.; Lip, G.Y.; Kamper, A.L.; Hommel, K.; Køber, L.; Lane, D.A.; Lindhardsen, J.; Gislason, G.H.; Torp-Pedersen, C. Stroke and bleeding in atrial fibrillation with chronic kidney disease. *N. Engl. J. Med.* **2012**, *367*, 625–635. [CrossRef]
21. Liao, J.N.; Chao, T.F.; Liu, C.J.; Wang, K.L.; Chen, S.J.; Lin, Y.J.; Chang, S.L.; Lo, L.W.; Hu, Y.F.; Tuan, T.C.; et al. Incidence and risk factors for new-onset atrial fibrillation among patients with end-stage renal disease undergoing renal replacement therapy. *Kidney Int.* **2015**, *87*, 1209–1215. [CrossRef]
22. Ocak, G.; Noordzij, M.; Rookmaaker, M.B.; Cases, A.; Couchoud, C.; Heaf, J.G.; Jarraya, F.; De Meester, J.; Groothoff, J.W.; Waldum-Grevbo, B.E.; et al. Mortality due to bleeding, myocardial infarction and stroke in dialysis patients. *J. Thromb. Haemost.* **2018**, *16*, 1953–1963. [CrossRef] [PubMed]
23. Shen, J.I.; Montez-Rath, M.E.; Lenihan, C.R.; Turakhia, M.P.; Chang, T.I.; Winkelmayer, W.C. Outcomes after warfarin initiation in a cohort of hemodialysis patients with newly diagnosed atrial fibrillation. *Am. J. Kidney Dis.* **2015**, *66*, 677–688. [CrossRef] [PubMed]
24. Kai, B.; Bogorad, Y.; Nguyen, L.N.; Yang, S.-J.; Chen, W.; Spencer, H.T.; Shen, A.Y.-J.; Lee, M.-S. Warfarin use and the risk of mortality, stroke, and bleeding in hemodialysis patients with atrial fibrillation. *Heart Rhythm* **2017**, *14*, 645–651. [CrossRef] [PubMed]
25. Heine, G.H.; Brandenburg, V.; Schirmer, S.H. Oral anticoagulation in chronic kidney disease and atrial fibrillation. *Dtsch. Arztebl. Int.* **2018**, *115*, 287–294. [CrossRef] [PubMed]
26. Akbar, M.R.; Febrianora, M.; Iqbal, M. Warfarin usage in patients with atrial fibrillation undergoing hemodialysis in the Indonesian population. *Curr. Probl. Cardiol.* **2023**, *48*, 101104. [CrossRef]
27. Lavalle, C.; Pierucci, N.; Mariani, M.V.; Piro, A.; Borrelli, A.; Grimaldi, M.; Rossillo, A.; Notarstefano, P.; Compagnucci, P.; Dello Russo, A.; et al. Italian Registry in the Setting of Atrial Fibrillation Ablation with Rivaroxaban—IRIS. *Minerva Cardiol. Angiol.* 2024, *ahead of print*. [CrossRef] [PubMed]
28. Cabanas-Grandio, P.; González-Melchor, L.; Caamaño, M.V.; Windcheid, E.F.-O.; Babarro, E.G.; Bobín, O.D.; Portela, M.P.; Delgado, O.P.; Teja, J.E.; Feijoo, M.G.; et al. Health-Related Quality of Life and Satisfaction in Atrial Fibrillation Patients on Anticoagulant Therapy: Differences between Vitamin K Antagonists and Direct Oral Anticoagulants; Results from the Multicentre REGUEIFA Registry. *J. Clin. Med.* **2024**, *13*, 5283. [CrossRef]
29. de Lucena, L.A.; Freitas, M.A.A.; Souza, A.K.C.; Silva, C.H.A.; Watanabe, J.M.F.; Guedes, F.L.; Almeida, J.B.; de Oliveira, R.A. Direct Oral Anticoagulants versus Vitamin K Antagonists in Patients with Atrial Fibrillation and Stage 5 Chronic Kidney Disease under Dialysis: A Systematic Review and Meta-Analysis of Randomized Controlled Trials. *J. Thromb. Thrombolysis* **2024**, *57*, 381–389. [CrossRef] [PubMed]

medicina

MDPI

Article

Vascular Access Type and Survival Outcomes in Hemodialysis Patients: A Seven-Year Cohort Study

Jesús Venegas-Ramírez [1], Gustavo A. Hernández-Fuentes [2,3,4], Claudia S. Palomares [5], Janet Diaz-Martinez [6], Joel I. Navarro-Cuellar [7], Patricia Calvo-Soto [8], Carlos Duran [9], Rosa Tapia-Vargas [10], Ana C. Espíritu-Mojarro [11], Alejandro Figueroa-Gutiérrez [12], José Guzmán-Esquivel [13], Daniel Antonio-Flores [14], Carmen Meza-Robles [3] and Iván Delgado-Enciso [2,3,15,*]

1 Department of Nephrology, Mexican Institute of Social Security (IMSS), General Hospital of Zone No. 1, IMSS, Villa de Alvarez 28984, Mexico; nefrojesusvr@gmail.com
2 Department of Molecular Medicine, School of Medicine, University of Colima, Colima 28040, Mexico; gahfuentes@gmail.com
3 State Cancerology Institute of Colima, Health Services of the Mexican Social Security Institute for Welfare (IMSS-BIENESTAR), Colima 28085, Mexico; carmen.qfb@gmail.com
4 Faculty of Chemical Sciences, University of Colima, Coquimatlan 28400, Mexico
5 Department of Internal Medicine, Mexican Institute of Social Security (IMSS), General Hospital of Zone No. 1, Villa de Alvarez 28984, Mexico; selenepacr@gmail.com
6 Department of Dietetics & Nutrition, Robert Stempel College of Public Health, Research Center in Minority Institutions, Florida International University, Miami, FL 33199, USA; jdimarti@fiu.edu
7 Department of Research, Mexican Institute of Social Security (IMSS), General Hospital of Zone No. 1, Villa de Alvarez 28984, Mexico; rosagonzalez@ucol.mx
8 Coordination of Planning and Institutional Liaison, IMSS OOAD Colima, Colima 28030, Mexico; patricia.calvo@imss.gob.mx
9 Florida Kidney Physicians, Boca Raton, FL 33431, USA; cmartinez@flkidney.com
10 Medical Education Auxiliary Coordination, Mexican Institute of Social Security (IMSS) OOAD Colima, Colima 28030, Mexico; rosa.tapia@imss.gob.mx
11 Department of Pediatrics, Mexican Institute of Social Security (IMSS), General Hospital of Zone No. 1, Villa de Alvarez 28984, Mexico; aespiritu3@ucol.mx
12 Health Education Auxiliary Coordination, Mexican Institute of Social Security (IMSS), Villa de Alvarez 28984, Mexico; alejandro.figueroag@imss.gob.mx
13 Clinical Epidemiology Research Unit, Mexican Institute of Social Security (IMSS), Villa de Alvarez 28984, Mexico; jose.esquivel@imss.gob.mx
14 Department of Nephrology, Mexican Institute of Social Security (IMSS), General Hospital of Zone No. 10, Manzanillo 28869, Mexico; restiforme@gmail.com
15 Robert Stempel College of Public Health and Social Work, Florida International University, Miami, FL 33199, USA
* Correspondence: ivan_delgado_enciso@ucol.mx; Tel./Fax: +52-312-3161099

Abstract: *Background and Objectives*: Arteriovenous fistulas (AVFs) are the preferred vascular access for hemodialysis due to their impact on patient outcomes, including survival, infection rates, and overall quality of life. Despite strong recommendations favoring AVF, gaps in AVF utilization remain, influenced by clinical, demographic, and systemic factors. This study is the first to analyze survival outcomes associated with different dialysis vascular access types, adjusting for key clinical, demographic variables, and other comorbidities over extended periods. *Materials and Methods*: This ambispective cohort study followed 428 hemodialysis patients over seven years. Patients were categorized based on their access type: AVF (n = 189), tunneled central venous catheter (CVC) (n = 178), and non-tunneled CVC (n = 61). Kaplan–Meier survival analysis was used to estimate survival curves, and Cox proportional hazards regression adjusted for potential confounders, including age, diabetes, and hypertension. *Results*: The 2-year survival rates were as follows: AVF 94.1%, tunneled CVC 70.0%, and non-tunneled CVC 36.6%. The 7-year survival rates were as follows: AVF 65.5%, tunneled CVC 26.4%, and non-tunneled CVC 11.0%. Compared to AVF, tunneled CVC use was associated with a 2.8-fold increased risk of mortality (adjusted hazard ratio [AdHR] 2.8, 95% CI 2.0–4.1), while non-tunneled CVC increased the risk 5-fold (AdHR 5.0, 95% CI 3.3–7.6). Notably, older adults, women, and diabetic patients were disproportionately represented in the groups with tunneled and non-tunneled catheters. *Conclusions*: Adjusted survival analyses highlight the significantly lower survival rates associated with CVC use compared to AVF. Non-tunneled catheters are generally not used for prolonged periods, and this cohort provides evidence of their prognosis for long-term use. These findings reinforce the need to prioritize AVF placement whenever feasible, reinforcing health education on this topic, to improve long-term outcomes for hemodialysis patients.

Keywords: hemodialysis; arteriovenous fistula; central venous catheter; survival analysis; cohort study; mortality risk; patient-centered care

1. Introduction

Chronic kidney disease (CKD) is a growing global public health concern, affecting more than 10% of the global population, with an estimated 800 million individuals living with the condition. CKD is progressive, and a significant proportion of patients advance to end-stage renal disease (ESRD), which requires renal replacement therapy such as hemodialysis (HD) to sustain life [1,2]. Globally, HD is the predominant modality of renal replacement therapy, utilized by 70% to 90% of ESRD patients, including nearly half a million individuals in the United States alone [1]. In Mexico, hemodialysis is the primary renal replacement therapy for patients with end-stage renal disease (ESRD), with a significant proportion relying on publicly funded healthcare institutions such as the Mexican Institute of Social Security (IMSS) and the Institute of Security and Social Services for State Workers (ISSSTE), as well as private providers [1,2]. IMSS alone provides renal replacement therapy to approximately 79,689 patients. However, access to hemodialysis services is often limited by geographic, economic, and infrastructural barriers, which results in disparities in treatment and outcomes [3,4]. The prevalence of ESRD in Mexico has been increasing, mainly due to high rates of diabetes and hypertension, the leading causes of chronic kidney disease (CKD) in the country [5].

Vascular access is crucial for HD patients, and the type of access plays a significant role in patients' outcomes, including survival and infection rates. There are two main types: arteriovenous (AV) access and central venous catheters (CVCs). AV access includes arteriovenous fistulas (AVFs) and arteriovenous grafts (AVGs), both of which are preferred over CVCs due to their superior long-term patency and lower complication rates [6,7]. Arteriovenous grafts (AVGs), however, have limited use in low- and middle-income countries. For example, in Mexico, recent studies showed that only 1.5% of patients used them, highlighting their rare utilization in clinical practice [8]. Despite strong recommendations favoring AVF as the preferred access, disparities in vascular access selection persist, influenced by clinical, demographic, and systemic factors [3,4].

AVF is considered the gold standard due to its superior long-term patency, significantly lower rates of thrombosis and infection, and reduced healthcare-related expenditures compared to AVG and CVC [5,6]. When successfully matured, AVF offers the best long-term outcomes for most HD patients, minimizing complications such as hospitalization and mortality [6,9]. Despite these well-documented advantages, their use remains suboptimal in many patient populations. CVCs, both tunneled and non-tunneled, are often employed as alternatives, particularly in patients with advanced age, multiple comorbidities, or anatomical challenges that may complicate fistula creation [10]. However, these catheters are associated with higher risks of bloodstream infections, thrombosis, and hospitalization, leading to poorer clinical outcomes [11,12]. In the United States, approximately 80% of patients initiate HD with a CVC [13,14]. In emergent or urgent dialysis situations, non-tunneled CVCs serve as a non-tunneled solution for managing conditions such as intoxications, uremic symptoms, or volume overload. Tunneled CVCs, most commonly placed in the internal jugular vein under imaging guidance, are preferred for longer-term use, ensuring the catheter tip resides in the mid-right atrium. Non-tunneled CVCs, inserted under ultrasound guidance, should be used only for short durations (up to two weeks) to minimize the risk of catheter-related infections. While CVCs are generally not ideal for long-term vascular access, they may be used tunneled in select cases when other options are not feasible [6,11].

International guidelines, such as the National Kidney Foundation–Kidney Disease Outcomes Quality Initiative (NKF-KDOQI) and the Fistula First Breakthrough Initiative in the United States (US), recommend prioritizing the use of AVFs over AVGs and aim to reduce reliance on CVCs [6,7]. Consequently, AVF use among long-term dialysis patients in the US increased from 32% in 2003 to 65% in 2014, while CVC use has concurrently declined [14]. However, despite these efforts, 80% of incident dialysis patients still initiate treatment with a catheter, and only one-quarter of these patients have a maturing AVF or AVG at the time of dialysis initiation [14]. While the United States has made progress in promoting AVF use [13,14], global disparities in vascular access utilization and success rates remain pronounced [10]. Findings from the Dialysis Outcomes and Practice Patterns Study (DOPPS) reveal substantial variations in AVF prevalence, ranging from over 90% in countries like Japan and Russia to just 49% in other regions [11]. Similarly, CVC dependence varies widely, with rates spanning 1% to 45% across different countries [12]. In Mexico, vascular access for hemodialysis varies significantly, with patients utilizing arteriovenous fistulas (AVFs), tunneled catheters, and non-tunneled catheters depending on healthcare availability and individual clinical conditions [12]. While AVFs are the preferred option due to their lower risk of infection and longer durability, their use remains suboptimal due to late nephrology referrals, limited surgical expertise, and delays in vascular access planning. These global differences in vascular access use reflect variations in healthcare infrastructure, surgical expertise, early CKD care, and vascular access planning, all of which continue to shape patient outcomes [15].

Beyond systemic and structural disparities, patient-level factors also play a crucial role in vascular access selection and outcomes [7]. Education, perceived benefits, and aesthetic concerns influence a patient's willingness to undergo AVF placement [16]. Barriers such as low health literacy, lack of disease awareness, and misperceptions about AVFs can further deter their acceptance [17]. Additionally, previous studies suggest that comorbidities such as diabetes and hypertension may significantly impact vascular access choice for HD [11,14]. Following AVF creation, several factors contribute to maturation failure, including age, vessel diameter, blood flow, and comorbidities like diabetes and cardiovascular disease [15]. The interplay between these physiological and patient-related factors underscores the complexity of vascular access selection across different patient populations, yet epidemiological studies on this subject remain scarce.

This study examines the distribution of vascular access types in a cohort of Mexican hemodialysis patients and analyzes the demographic and clinical characteristics associated with access selection and its implications for survival. It explores how factors, such as age, sex, diabetes, and hypertension, influence vascular access choice and mortality risk. By providing a deeper understanding of the factors shaping vascular access selection and related outcomes, this research contributes to the broader discourse on patient-centered hemodialysis care, optimization of vascular access practices, and improved clinical outcomes.

2. Materials and Methods

2.1. Study Design and Setting

This ambispective cohort study was conducted between 2018 and 2023 at a single tertiary care center specializing in hemodialysis (General Hospital Zone 1 of the Mexican Social Security; Colima, Mexico). The study followed patients over a maximum period of 7 years to evaluate the association between vascular access types and long-term survival. The three vascular access types included arteriovenous (A-V) fistulas, tunneled catheters, and non-tunneled catheters. Relevant clinical risk factors were adjusted to provide a comprehensive analysis of patient outcomes.

2.2. Participants

This study included adult patients undergoing hemodialysis, selected based on specific inclusion and exclusion criteria. Participants were eligible for inclusion if they were 18 years of age or older and received regular hemodialysis treatment using one of the predefined vascular access types (arteriovenous fistula, tunneled catheter). Patients with AVGs were not included, as this type of vascular access is rarely used in the analyzed healthcare institution (only four patients during the study period). Those with incomplete clinical records were excluded, as were individuals lost to follow-up before the study's conclusion. Careful screening ensured that the final cohort comprised only patients with comprehensive data and consistent follow-up, enhancing the reliability of the study findings. Additionally, patients who survived during the follow-up period but had less than seven years of follow-up were excluded, along with those who were lost to follow-up. A total of 428 patients were included in the analysis after excluding 211 living patients who did not complete the minimum follow-up period and 40 patients lost to follow-up (28 with tunneled catheters, 11 with AVFs, and 1 with a temporary catheter) (see Figure 1).

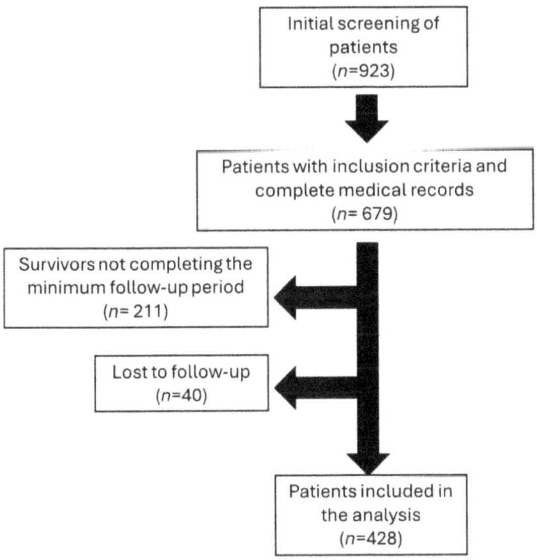

Figure 1. Flowchart of patient selection and characteristics for hemodialysis analysis.

2.3. Variables

The primary exposure variable in this study was the type of vascular access used for hemodialysis, which included arteriovenous fistulas, tunneled catheters, and non-tunneled catheters. An arteriovenous fistula (AVF) is a surgically created connection between an artery and a vein, usually in the arm, and is considered the gold standard for vascular access. AVFs are preferred due to their superior long-term patency, lower risks of infection and thrombosis, and their association with improved survival rates [18]. Tunneled catheters, on the other hand, are tunneled devices inserted into large central veins, such as the internal jugular or subclavian vein, and are designed for long-term use [19]. Although they are a viable alternative for patients who cannot undergo AVF creation, tunneled catheters carry significantly higher risks of bloodstream infections, thrombosis, and other complications. Non-tunneled catheters are typically placed for short-term use and are inserted percutaneously into central veins [20]. While they are often used as an immediate solution for vascular access, non-tunneled catheters are associated with the highest risks of infection, thrombosis, and adverse outcomes, making them unsuitable for long-term hemodialysis. The primary outcome of this study was overall survival (OS) over a 7-year follow-up period. Covariates included demographic and clinical factors, such as age, gender (male or female, based on official identification), diabetes mellitus (diagnosed based on medical history or the use of hypoglycemic agents), and hypertension (defined as a history of blood pressure > 140/90 mmHg or the use of antihypertensive medication). Other covariates included hospitalization (defined as any hospital admission lasting more than 24 h), sepsis (documented systemic infection requiring antimicrobial treatment during follow-up), myocardial infarction (MI) (diagnosed based on clinical, biochemical, and electrocardiographic criteria), and cerebrovascular disease (CVD) (defined as a history of ischemic or hemorrhagic stroke confirmed by imaging or clinical evaluation).

2.4. Data Collection

Patient data were collected from the institutional electronic medical records, where demographic, clinical, and laboratory information was extracted. This included details about the type of vascular access, comorbidities, and patient outcomes, such as mortality and hospitalizations. To ensure accuracy, the survival status of all patients was verified through hospital records, and when necessary, follow-up was conducted via telephone.

2.5. Ethical Considerations

The study protocol was reviewed and approved by the local health research committee of IMSS-Colima, Mexico, under approval number R-2018-785-056 on 12 June 2018. Informed consent was waived as the data were obtained retrospectively from clinical records and not directly from patients. All data were anonymized to protect patient confidentiality. This study adhered to the ethical principles outlined in the Declaration of Helsinki, maintaining strict confidentiality and data security throughout the research process [21].

2.6. Sample Size and Power Calculation

The sample size was estimated based on the survival differences observed between vascular access types over a 2-year period [22], as reported in previous studies [6], where survival with an AVF was 69%, compared to 38% with a catheter. Using a significance level (α) of 0.05 and a statistical power (1-β) of 80%, the required sample size for comparing the groups with the largest survival contrasts was calculated to be 39 patients per group. Upon completion of this study, a post hoc statistical power analysis was conducted. The analysis revealed that having an AVF significantly reduced mortality in hemodialysis patients after 7 years of follow-up. The statistical power for this finding was 99.9% when compared to the tunneled catheter group and 99.9% when compared to the non-tunneled catheter group.

2.7. Statistical Analysis

Continuous variables were reported as means with their corresponding standard deviations (SD), while categorical variables were summarized as counts and percentages.

Group comparisons were performed using Fisher's exact test for qualitative variables, while ANOVA or Student's *t*-test was used for quantitative data, as appropriate [23]. The normality of the data distribution was verified using the Kolmogorov–Smirnov test. Survival outcomes over a 7-year period were assessed for a cohort of 428 patients using the Kaplan–Meier method for survival analysis. To identify independent risk factors for overall survival, univariate and multivariate Cox proportional hazards regression analyses were conducted, generating hazard ratios (HRs), which were interpreted as measures of relative risk [24]. The predictors of significant outcomes were determined and subsequently examined in a multivariable model. A forward stepwise Cox regression was then used to identify the most efficient model. For the stepwise regression, a variable entry threshold of 0.05 and a removal threshold of 0.10 were applied. The vascular access route (AVF, tunneled catheter, or non-tunneled catheter) was incorporated into the model as a 'stratum' only when analyzing the risk of covariates. The Omnibus Tests of Model Coefficients were used to evaluate whether the inclusion of explanatory variables significantly improved the baseline survival model. A chi-square test was employed to compare the log-likelihoods of the baseline and updated models, assessing significant differences [25]. The concordance index (C-index) was calculated to assess the predictive ability of the multivariate Cox regression models. The C-index was calculated using R software (ver. 4.4.1). The adjusted survival curve, derived from the Cox Proportional Hazards Model, was graphically displayed, representing the survival function at the mean of the covariates [25,26]. All statistical analyses were conducted using SPSS version 25 (IBM Corp., Armonk, NY, USA), except for statistical power and sample size, which were calculated using ClinCalc version 1 (https://clincalc.com/stats/Power.aspx, accessed on 15 January 2025) [27,28]. A significance level of $p < 0.05$ was considered statistically significant.

3. Results

3.1. General Characteristics

Initially, 923 patients were screened, of whom only 679 were included because they had a complete medical record. After the evaluation period was over, 211 survivors were eliminated because they did not complete the minimum follow-up period required, which was 7 years. Forty patients were lost to follow-up. A total of 428 patients on hemodialysis were included in the analysis (Figure 1), with the majority having a tunneled catheter (53.0%, $n = 227$), followed by AVF (27.8%, $n = 119$) and non-tunneled catheter (19.2%, $n = 82$). The average age was 58.39 years (SD 15.53), with 38.6% of patients being women. Age was significantly lower in patients with AVF (51.75 years, SD 15.59) compared to those with a tunneled catheter (60.78 years, SD 14.99, $p < 0.001$) or non-tunneled catheter (61.43 years, SD 14.13, $p < 0.001$).

Table 1 shows that women, patients aged 60 years or older, and those with diabetes were significantly more likely to have a tunneled or non-tunneled catheter, compared to those with an AVF ($p < 0.05$ for all comparisons, see Table 1). It can be observed that patients with AVFs had fewer occurrences of sepsis and hospitalizations (see Table 1). Notably, after 7 years of follow-up, the group with AVF had the lowest mortality rate (34.5%), which was significantly lower than the mortality rates of those with a tunneled catheter (73.6%, $p < 0.001$) and non-tunneled catheter (89.0%, $p < 0.001$) (see Table 1).

Table 1. Comparison of key clinical characteristics of hemodialysis patients based on vascular access route.

Variable	All Patients 100% (428)	Catheter			p-Value *			
		Fistula A-V 27.8% (119)	Tunneled 53.0% (227)	Temporal 19.2% (82)	Inter-Group	F vs. P	F vs. T	P vs. T
>60 years	52.6% (225)	33.6% (40)	59.5% (135)	61.0% (50)	<0.001	<0.001	<0.001	0.896
Female	38.6% (165)	26.1% (31)	42.7% (97)	45.1% (37)	0.003	0.002	0.006	0.795
Diabetes	59.8% (256)	42.9% (51)	63.4% (144)	74.4% (61)	<0.001	<0.001	<0.001	0.078
Hypertension (HTA)	80.4% (344)	84.0% (100)	80.6% (183)	74.4% (61)	0.245	0.467	0.107	0.269
Hospitalizations	23.6% (101)	13.4% (16)	25.6% (58)	32.9% (27)	0.003	0.009	0.001	0.248
Acute Myocardial Infarction (AMI)	7.2% (31)	9.2% (11)	6.2% (14)	7.3% (6)	0.587	0.382	0.798	0.794
Stroke (EVC)	5.60% (24)	3.40% (4)	5.30% (12)	9.80% (8)	0.168	0.592	0.073	0.190
Sepsis	12.1% (52)	6.7% (8)	15.9% (369	9.8% (8)	0.03	0.017	0.441	0.201
Mortality	65.7% (281)	34.5% (41)	73.6% (167)	89.0% (73)	<0.001	<0.001	<0.001	0.003

* To compare three groups (intergroup analysis), or to compare two groups, Fisher's exact test was used. F = Fistula A-V. P = Tunneled. T = Temporal.

3.2. Effect of Vascular Access Types on Survival

In a 7-year (84 months) survival follow-up (Kaplan–Meier curves), significant differences were observed among the various vascular access types for dialysis ($p < 0.001$, multigroup log-rank test). Individuals with an AVF exhibited a higher survival rate (mean 72.4 months, 95% CI 68.7–76.2, survivors 65.5%), while those with a non-tunneled catheter had a lower survival rate (mean 25.9 months, 95% CI 20.4–31.4, survivors 11.0%), with individuals with a tunneled catheter falling in between (mean 46.8 months, 95% CI 43.1–50.6, survivors 26.4%) (see Figure 2 and Table 2).

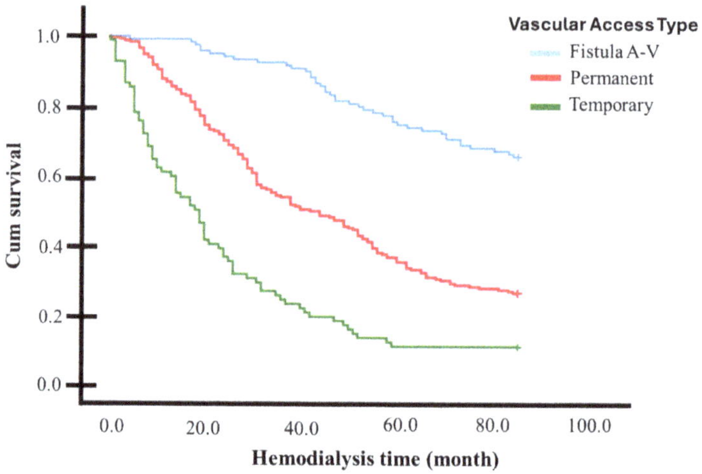

Figure 2. Kaplan–Meier curves for 84-month follow-up (7 Years) based on vascular access for dialysis: individuals with an AVF exhibited a higher survival rate than those with tunneled and non-tunneled catheters ($p < 0.001$, multigroup log-rank test).

Table 2. Overall survival of hemodialysis patients in 84-month follow-up (7 years), according to vascular access route.

	Survival Rate At			Survival Time		
	2 Years	5 Years	7 Years	Months	95% CI	
Global	70.3%	41.6%	34.3%	49.9	47.0	52.8
Fistula A-V	94.1%	74.8%	65.5%	72.4	68.7	76.2

Table 2. *Cont.*

	Survival Rate At			Survival Time		
	2 Years	5 Years	7 Years	Months	95% CI	
Tunneled	70.0%	35.2%	26.4%	46.8	43.1	50.6
Non-tunneled	36.6%	11.0%	11.0%	25.9	20.4	31.4
p-value intergroup	<0.001	<0.001	<0.001	<0.001		
p-value (F vs. P)	<0.001	<0.001	<0.001	<0.001		
p-value (F vs. T)	<0.001	<0.001	<0.001	<0.001		
p-value (P vs. T)	<0.001	<0.001	<0.001	<0.001		

F = Fistula A-V. P = Tunneled. T = Temporal.

3.3. Adjusted Overall Survival According to the Presence of Other Risk Factors

The overall survival (OS) information based on the Cox Proportional Risk Model is provided in Tables 3 and 4. The independent variables included in the model are as follows: age (>60 years), gender, history of diabetes, hypertension, hospitalization, sepsis, acute myocardial infarction (AMI), and stroke (EVC). Table 3 shows the collective controls for adjusting the reciprocal model. Since the χ^2 variation is statistically significant ($p < 0.001$), the model is well adjusted, meaning that at least one of the independent variables significantly affects survival time (see Table 3).

Table 3. Omnibus tests of model coefficients.

	Overall (Score)			Change from Previous Step			Change from Previous Block		
−2 Loglikelihood	χ^2	Df	Sig.	χ^2	df	Sig.	χ^2	df	Sig.
2469.930	92.166	8	<0.001	90.201	8	<0.001	90.201	8	<0.001

df: Degrees of freedom; Sig.: Statistical significance.

Table 4. Univariate and multivariate cox regression model for overall survival in 7-year follow-up.

	Unadjusted	95% CI			Adjusted	95% CI		
Covariate	HR	Lower	Upper	*p*	HR	Lower	Upper	*p*
Age > 60 years	1.881	1.464	2.418	<0.001	1.345	1.032	1.752	0.028
Female	1.130	0.890	1.435	0.317				
Diabetic	2.428	1.845	3.196	<0.001	2.393	1.784	3.210	<0.001
Hypertension (HTA)	0.549	0.418	0.721	<0.001	0.474	0.358	0.627	<0.001
Hospitalization	1.467	1.134	1.899	0.004	1.654	1.274	2.146	<0.001
Sepsis	1.002	0.715	1.404	0.990				
Acute Myocardial Infarction (AMI)	1.022	0.648	1.613	0.956				
Stroke (EVC)	0.923	0.570	1.495	0.744				

The predictors of significant outcomes were determined (univariate model) (unadjusted HR) and subsequently examined in a multivariable model (adjusted HR). Forward stepwise Cox regression was then used to identify the most efficient model. For the stepwise regression, a variable entry threshold of 0.05 and a removal threshold of 0.10 were applied. The vascular access route (AVF, tunneled catheter, or non-tunneled catheter) was incorporated into the model as "strata".

Table 4 presents the hazard ratios (HRs) obtained from the univariate and multivariate Cox regression models. The types of vascular access for hemodialysis were all considered as strata. Across 84 months (7 years) of hemodialysis, being diabetic (AdHR 2.38, 95% CI 1.77–3.20) or having been hospitalized (AdHR 1.80, 95% CI 1.36–2.38) approximately doubles the risk of death, while having a history of hypertension reduces this risk by half (AdHR 0.45, 95% CI 0.34–0.60). Being 60 years or older increases the likelihood of death by 37% during the follow-up period compared to those younger than 60 years (AdHR

1.374, 95% CI 1.052–1.795). Since these three factors frequently occur together, interactions between them were analyzed in independent multivariate models. The joint presence of diabetes and hypertension nullified the risk modification presented by each of these variables separately (AdHR 1.218, 95% CI 0.949–1.562, $p = 0.122$), as did having hypertension and being 60 years or older (AdHR 1.067, 95% CI 0.828–1.373, $p = 0.617$). Simultaneously having diabetes and being 60 years or older (AdHR 2.006, 95% CI 1.574–2.557, $p < 0.001$), or having diabetes and being hospitalized (AdHR 2.215, 95% CI 1.633–3.004, $p < 0.001$), or being 60 years or older and hospitalized (AdHR 1.825, 95% CI 1.309–2.544, $p < 0.001$), did not substantially modify the risk generated by diabetes or hospitalization alone. The protective factor of having a history of hypertension disappears in patients who have been hospitalized, with an elevated risk of death when these two factors occur together (AdHR 1.567, 95% CI 1.187–2.069, $p = 0.002$). A statistical model that included all the adjustment variables listed in Table 4 determined that having a tunneled catheter increased the probability of death 2.8-times in the 7-year follow-up period, compared with AVF (AdHR 2.892, 95% CI 2.036–4.108, $p < 0.001$). On the other hand, the use of a non-tunneled catheter increased the probability of death 5-times compared with AVF (AdHR 5.047, 95% CI 3.333–7.643, $p < 0.001$). In terms of model performance, the concordance index (C-index) for the tunneled catheter model was 0.684, reflecting reasonable discriminatory ability to differentiate between patients who experienced death and those who did not over the 7-year follow-up period. In comparison, the C-index for the non-tunneled catheter model was 0.768, suggesting a slightly better discriminatory ability. These values indicate that both models demonstrate good overall predictive accuracy. The adjusted survival curve (based on the Cox Proportional Risk Model) is graphically presented in Figure 3.

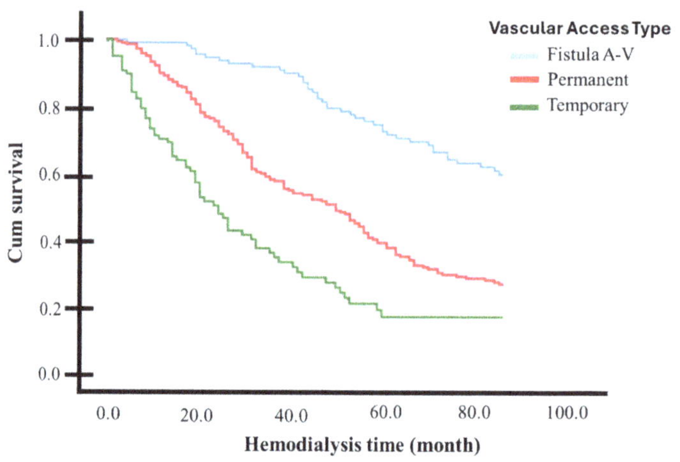

Figure 3. Adjusted survival curves for patients with or without significant risk factors identified. Log-rank test ($p < 0.05$).

3.4. Survival Based on the Presence or Absence of Risk Factors

The 7-year survival rates of hemodialysis patients were analyzed according to the presence or absence of identified risk factors (see Table 3). Table 5 demonstrates that age >60 years, diabetes, hypertension, and hospitalization significantly impact survival rates across the entire cohort, particularly in patients with AVFs and tunneled catheters (see Table 4). However, in patients with non-tunneled catheters, no significant differences in 7-year survival rates were observed based on these risk factors, likely due to the low frequency of patients surviving this period. Across the entire cohort, only 18.4% of diabetic patients survived 7 years, compared to 58.1% of non-diabetic patients. Vascular access type significantly influenced these outcomes. Among patients with AVFs, 41.2% of diabetics and 83.8% of non-diabetics survived ($p < 0.001$). In contrast, among patients with non-tunneled catheters, only 8.2% of diabetics and 19.0% of non-diabetics survived ($p < 0.001$). Detailed survival percentages for all strata are provided in Table 4. Figure 4 presents the adjusted survival curves for patients with or without each of the significant risk factors identified in this study.

Table 5. Overall survival during a 7-year follow-up according to the presence or absence of risk factors and the type of vascular access.

Variable (Factor)	Patients (*n*)	Factor Presence	Vascular Access Type			
			Global (*n* = 428)	AVF (*n* = 119)	Tunneled (*n* = 227)	Non-Tunneled (*n* = 82)
>60 years old	203	No	51.20%	73.40%	43.50%	18.80%
	225	Yes	19.10%	50.00%	14.80%	6.00%
p-value *			<0.001	0.015	<0.001	0.144
Diabetes	172	No	58.10%	83.80%	47.00%	19.00%
	256	Yes	18.40%	41.20%	14.60%	8.20%
p-value *			<0.001	<0.001	<0.001	0.224
Hypertension	84	No	16.70%	36.80%	13.60%	4.80%
	344	Yes	38.70%	71.00%	29.50%	13.10%
p-value *			<0.001	0.007	0.036	0.435
Hospitalization	327	No	40.4%	70.9%	30.8%	12.7%
	101	Yes	14.90%	31.30%	13.80%	7.40%
p-value *			<0.001	0.004	0.015	0.711

* *p*-value: Comparison of survival rates between "Yes" and "No" for each variable in each vascular access stratum.

The survival function at the mean of covariates is presented according to vascular access type and the presence or absence of risk factors that significantly affect survival, as shown in Tables 3 and 4. The curves demonstrate that being diabetic (A), not having hypertension, being aged 60 years or older, and having been hospitalized are factors associated with reduced survival over time. The Figure 4 clearly illustrates the cumulative impact of these factors on overall survival, highlighting the differences across vascular access types and patient risk profiles.

To identify interactions between variables, we analyzed the stratum-specific effects of various factors. Effect modification, which involves stratification, occurs when an exposure produces different effects across subgroups. This approach includes visually inspecting the data to identify patterns of variation in stratum-specific estimates. If these estimates remain consistent, it suggests no interaction, whereas discrepancies indicate the presence of an interaction, highlighting how the association of interest is influenced by the stratifying factor. It is important to note that while stratum-specific effect modification is useful for exploring and suggesting potential interactions, effect modification can occur without interaction, and interaction can exist without effect modification [29–31].

We conducted a stratified analysis by categorizing the study population into subgroups based on significant clinical variables identified in the prior multivariate analysis (Table 4). This method enabled the investigation of effect modification (AdHR) on mortality, with AVF serving as the reference category (see Table 6). It can be observed that a modification effect exists, meaning changes in the AdHR based on the presence or absence of being 60 years or older, hypertension, diabetes, or a history of hospitalization. This pertains to the increased mortality associated with having a tunneled or non-tunneled catheter compared to AVF (reference). A significant difference is highlighted between the diabetes strata, where having a non-tunneled vascular access increases the probability of death by 10-times over 7 years compared to AVF (AdHR 10.024, 95% CI 4.351–23.098), whereas in diabetic individuals, the probability of death was only 4-times higher compared to AVF (AdHR 4.418, 95% CI 2.752–7.093) (Table 6).

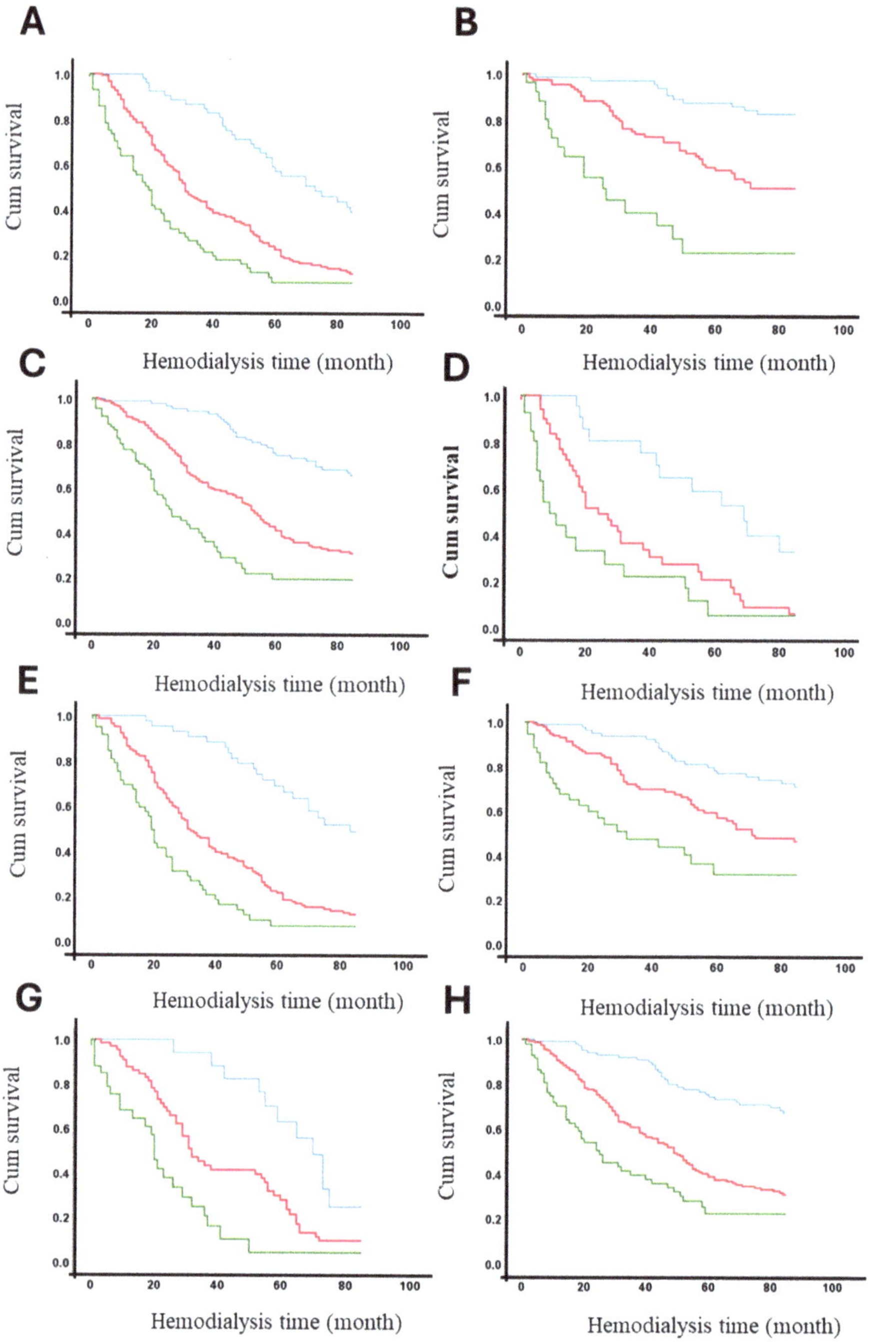

Figure 4. Adjusted survival curves (in months) based on vascular access and the presence or absence of significant risk factors. Panels represent survival stratified by different conditions: (**A**) diabetic patients, (**B**) non-diabetic patients, (**C**) hypertensive patients, (**D**) non-hypertensive patients, (**E**) patients aged $\geq$ 60 years, (**F**) patients aged < 60 years, (**G**) patients with hospitalization, and (**H**) patients without hospitalization. Vascular Access Type: AVF (blue line), Permanent (red line) and Temporary (green line).

Table 6. Stratum-specific effects on 7-year mortality risk with the use of tunneled and non-tunneled catheters compared to arteriovenous fistulas.

Factor Presence	No				Yes			
	AdHR	Lower	Upper	*p*	AdHR	Lower	Upper	*p*
All								
AVF	1 (Baseline value)							
Tunneled	2.892	2.036	4.108	<0.001				
Non-tunneled	5.047	3.333	7.643	<0.001				
≥60 years old								
AVF	1 (baseline value)				1 (baseline value)			
Tunneled	2.261	1.344	3.806	0.002	3.132	1.939	5.059	<0.001
Non-tunneled	4.570	2.425	8.613	<0.001	6.276	3.473	11.342	<0.001
Diabetes								
AVF	1 (baseline value)				1 (baseline value)			
Tunneled	3.416	1.734	6.729	<0.001	2.603	1.735	3.905	<0.001
Non-tunneled	10.024	4.351	23.098	<0.001	4.418	2.752	7.093	<0.001
Hypertension								
AVF	1 (baseline value)				1 (baseline value)			
Tunneled	2.618	1.346	5.092	<0.001	2.857	1.896	4.306	<0.001
Non-tunneled	4.319	1.981	9.415	<0.001	5.531	3.380	9.051	<0.001
Hospitalization								
AVF	1 (baseline value)				1 (baseline value)			
Tunneled	2.920	1.940	4.397	<0.001	2.449	1.260	4.761	0.008
Non-tunneled	5.223	3.170	8.606	<0.001	7.814	3.063	19.936	<0.001

Multivariate Cox proportional hazards regression analyses were performed. In different strata (Presence of the Factor: No or Yes), the 7-year mortality risk was calculated for the vascular access route (tunneled catheter or non-tunneled catheter), with AVF as the baseline value (HR = 1). The variables of being 60 years or older, diabetes, hypertension, and a history of hospitalization were included as covariates for all analyses.

4. Discussion

This study provides a comprehensive evaluation of the long-term impact of vascular access type on overall survival among hemodialysis (HD) patients, with a seven-year follow-up period. To our knowledge, this is one of the most extensive studies to analyze survival differences among patients using arteriovenous fistulas (AVFs), tunneled catheters, and non-tunneled catheters, while accounting for comorbidities and clinical risk factors in a high-risk population. Our findings demonstrate that patients with AVFs had the highest survival rates, with a 65.5% survival rate at seven years, compared to 26.4% for tunneled catheter users and 11.0% for non-tunneled catheter users. The use of both non-tunneled and tunneled catheters was associated with significantly reduced survival rates compared to AVFs, reinforcing their limited suitability for long-term HD.

These results align with global guidelines and recommendations, which emphasize the critical role of optimal vascular access in determining long-term survival among patients undergoing HD [32]. In addition, our findings also highlight the modulating effects of clinical and demographic factors on vascular access outcomes, particularly age, diabetes, hypertension, and hospitalization. Consistent with prior studies, diabetes and hospitalization were strongly associated with an increased mortality risk [6], whereas hypertension appeared to have a protective effect when considered in isolation. This seemingly paradoxical finding aligns with the concept of "reverse epidemiology" in dialysis patients, where traditional cardiovascular risk factors, such as hypertension and higher body mass index, have been linked to improved survival outcomes in this population [33,34]. Several physiological mechanisms have been proposed to explain this phenomenon, including the potential role of higher blood pressure in maintaining adequate perfusion of the arteriovenous fistula (AVF) and preventing access failure. Additionally, hypertension has been associated with a higher likelihood of successful AVF maturation, which could contribute to improved long-term vascular access patency and, consequently, better survival outcomes [35]. However, while hypertension may appear protective in this context, it is important to interpret these findings with caution. The long-term effects of poorly controlled hypertension on cardiovascular health, arterial stiffness, and vascular complications remain a concern [36]. Further research is needed to better understand the balance between its potential short-term benefits and long-term risks in hemodialysis patients [37]. These observations underscore the complex interplay between patient comorbidities and vascular access outcomes, emphasizing the need for individualized vascular access planning in high-risk populations with multiple comorbidities.

Interestingly, the survival advantage conferred by AVF remained robust even in the presence of adverse risk factors, including diabetes and advanced age. The protective effect of AVF persisted after adjusting for multiple risk factors, as demonstrated by Cox proportional hazards modeling. The survival benefits associated with AVF were consistent across all subgroups, even among patients with significant comorbidities such as diabetes. For instance, among diabetic patients, those with AVF had a survival rate of 41.2% after seven years, compared to 14.6% for those with tunneled catheters and 8.2% for those with non-tunneled catheters. These findings emphasize the importance of prioritizing AVF placement, particularly in high-risk populations such as diabetic patients. However, our study also revealed that the survival advantage of AVF was less pronounced in older adults, especially when combined with diabetes or frequent hospitalizations [32]. This suggests that the benefits of superior vascular access may be partially offset by comorbidities and complications associated with aging, highlighting the need for individualized treatment plans in older HD patients. In contrast, the already-poor survival outcomes associated with tunneled and non-tunneled catheters were further exacerbated by risk factors such as diabetes and advanced age. An important factor that may influence the mortality of patients with CVC is catheter-related infection. A recent meta-analysis examined the impact of managing these infections and suggested that appropriate treatment could improve survival [38]. While reduced Kt/V is generally associated with higher mortality, infections may also play a crucial role in patient outcomes. Therefore, proper infection management should be considered in future studies and clinical strategies to enhance patient survival [38].

These findings reinforce the urgent need to minimize catheter use and to transition patients with tunneled catheters to AVF whenever feasible, particularly in those with comorbid conditions that further compromise survival. The survival advantage of AVF observed in this study aligns with prior research, which has consistently established AVF as the preferred vascular access for hemodialysis due to its lower risks of complications, including infections, thrombosis, and other adverse events [17,25,26,39]. Conversely, the high mortality rates observed in patients with tunneled and non-tunneled catheters reflect the significant risks associated with catheter use, particularly catheter-related bloodstream infections (CRBSIs) and poor hemodynamic performance [28,32,40].

These findings have significant implications for clinical practice and health policy. They reinforce KDOQI recommendations to prioritize AVF as the preferred vascular access for chronic HD patients [40] and emphasize the need for early referrals to vascular surgery to ensure timely fistula creation, particularly in high-risk patients such as those with diabetes. This study also underscores the urgency of minimizing catheter use and transitioning patients to AVF whenever possible, especially those with comorbidities that compromise survival. Additionally, the observed interplay between comorbidities and vascular access type highlights the need for a patient-centered approach in vascular access planning.

Beyond vascular access type, this study identified several independent clinical predictors of survival. Diabetes mellitus increased the mortality risk by 2.38-times, while hospitalizations elevated it by 1.80-times, consistent with previous studies. Advanced age ($\geq$60 years) was also associated with a 37% higher mortality risk. Interestingly, hypertension, traditionally considered a cardiovascular risk factor, appeared to have a protective effect, reducing the mortality risk by 55%. This aligns with the concept of "reverse epidemiology" observed in dialysis populations, where higher blood pressure may confer survival benefits under certain clinical conditions [35,39]. Given the well-established impact of diabetes on mortality in HD patients [41], addressing modifiable risk factors, such as diabetes control and infection prevention, remains essential for improving long-term outcomes in this high-risk population [26].

The analysis of our data raises critical concerns about potential disparities in access to optimal vascular modalities, particularly AVF placement. Older adults, women, and diabetic patients were disproportionately represented in the groups with tunneled and non-tunneled catheters, while AVF recipients were significantly younger, with a mean age of 51.75 years, compared to 60.78 years for tunneled catheter users and 61.43 years for non-tunneled catheter users. These patterns may suggest the presence of implicit biases or structural barriers that may inadvertently disadvantage certain populations, preventing them from accessing the survival benefits associated with AVF. Zarkowsky et al. (2015) [42] also reported that being female, of Black race, or having peripheral arterial disease reduced the probability of starting hemodialysis with an AVF. Additionally, their findings indicated that hypertension was linked to a higher likelihood of successful AVF maturation at the initiation of dialysis. Like our study, they found that diabetes negatively impacted AVF maturation.

Several other factors may contribute to these disparities. Physicians may prioritize AVF placement in younger patients, assuming a better long-term prognosis, which could unintentionally disadvantage older adults [34]. Similarly, anatomical differences in women or higher surgical risks in diabetic patients may influence clinical decision making, despite evidence supporting the long-term benefits of AVF in these populations [40,41]. Additionally, socioeconomic barriers, limited access to specialized care, and inadequate patient education about vascular access options may further contribute to these inequities [13].

It is essential to recognize the barriers at the patient, physician, and systemic levels that hinder timely referral for preoperative vein mapping, AVF placement, and maturation. These challenges are often exacerbated by delays in nephrology care before dialysis initiation [13,14]. Additionally, the unpredictable progression of CKD to ESRD and the variability in dialysis initiation thresholds further complicate timely vascular access planning. Some patients may also experience denial or reluctance to undergo vascular placement, opting instead for immediate but suboptimal solutions, such as tunneled and non-tunneled catheters, which prioritize clinical expediency over long-term benefits [43,44].

Addressing these challenges, particularly for older adults, women, and diabetic patients, requires early nephrology referral, structural interventions, and comprehensive patient education to ensure equitable access to optimal vascular care. All patients, regardless of demographic or clinical factors, must be informed about the survival and outcome advantages of AVF, enabling them to make informed decisions about their treatment. CKD education during stages 4 and 5 should cover dialysis modalities and tunneled vascular access options, emphasizing the long-term benefits of AVF [45]. Additionally, equitable clinical decision making and tailored interventions, such as educational programs for both patients and providers, are essential to reinforcing the benefits of AVF across all demographic groups [43]. Future research should explore whether vascular access selection patterns reflect clinical necessity or systemic inequities and further investigate the impact of socioeconomic status and healthcare access on decision making.

Education on the importance of arteriovenous fistula (AVF) inclusion in vascular access decisions is crucial, particularly as patients may not fully understand its long-term benefits. In some cases, the decision to forego AVF is influenced by convenience, lack of adequate information, or misconceptions about the procedure [46,47]. Additionally, family members, who often accompany patients to consultations, play a significant role in the decision-making process. Their perceptions and concerns, whether based on limited knowledge or cultural factors, can impact the patient's choices regarding vascular access options. Therefore, comprehensive education that includes both patients and their families is essential to ensure that AVF is considered as a primary option for vascular access, empowering patients to make informed decisions that optimize their long-term health outcomes [48].

Interdisciplinary care has emerged as an effective alternative to traditional nephrology care, enhancing patient education, health outcomes, and tunneled access placement. Studies from the United States, Taiwan, and Canada demonstrate that multidisciplinary care improves vascular access outcomes. Patients in interdisciplinary CKD clinics, who were more likely to start dialysis with tunneled vascular access rather than a catheter [49, 50], had lower CVC use [51] and experienced fewer urgent dialysis starts [52]. These findings highlight the importance of team-based approaches in optimizing vascular access and patient outcomes. It is important to note that patient preferences and physician guidance play a significant role in the selection of vascular access and can influence survival outcomes [44]. Patients often make decisions based on personal factors, such as previous experiences, perceived quality of life, and the potential risks and benefits of each access type [53]. For example, some patients may prefer a certain type of access due to concerns about comfort, long-term care, or aesthetic considerations [17]. On the other hand, physicians, based on their clinical expertise, guide patients toward the most appropriate vascular access choice considering individual factors such as comorbidities, anatomy, and expected complications [44]. The alignment of patient preferences with physician recommendations in regard to the sociocultural environment of the patient can positively impact adherence and satisfaction, which, in turn, may enhance the success of the chosen vascular access [54]. A more in-depth exploration of these factors could provide valuable insights into how decision-making processes, influenced by both patient preferences and physician guidance, affect long-term outcomes in hemodialysis patients. In addition to this, it is important to take care of the pre-ESRD care as a key factor in vascular access decisions. It is important to note that in Mexico, this service is typically available within hemodialysis units. In our study, all patients, regardless of vascular access type, received the same pre-ESRD planning, health education, and guidance before requiring hemodialysis. As IMSS beneficiaries in Colima, they were treated at the same medical center, minimizing differences in outcomes due to prior education. However, our study did not include specific pre-ESRD care data. While this factor could influence access decisions, the institution lacked a dedicated educational program for kidney disease, representing an area for improvement around the world [55]. Previous reports highlight delays in implementing a national renal health program in Mexico [56]. Our research focused on vascular access outcomes in hemodialysis patients, but future studies should explore the impact of pre-ESRD care on access selection and prognosis.

Our study has several limitations. First, as with all observational studies, patients were not randomly assigned to different vascular access groups, making the study susceptible to selection bias. Patients typically receive vascular access based on clinical decisions, which may be influenced by their individual characteristics, such as comorbidities or disease severity. This can lead to differences in outcomes that are not solely attributable to the type of vascular access but, rather, to the underlying health status of the patients. Despite adjusting for multiple covariates, residual confounding cannot be entirely ruled out. Second, another limitation is the single-center nature of this study, which may restrict the generalizability of our findings to other healthcare settings with different resources, patient demographics, or clinical practices. Future multicenter studies with more diverse populations are needed to validate these results and provide a broader understanding of vascular access selection and outcomes. Third, we lacked formal assessments of patient preferences and clinical staff proficiency, preventing us from exploring their potential influence on vascular access selection and long-term outcomes. Future research incorporating qualitative methodologies could offer valuable insights into how patient perceptions, health literacy, and clinician decision making impact vascular access choices. Finally, we did not evaluate socioeconomic factors and healthcare accessibility, which could play a significant role in vascular access selection and patient outcomes. Future studies should consider these aspects to provide a more comprehensive perspective.

Notwithstanding these limitations, our study has several notable strengths. The ambispective cohort design, large sample size, and long-term follow-up period enhance the study's robustness and reliability. The use of multivariate Cox regression analysis allowed for rigorous adjustment for potential confounders, strengthening the validity of our findings. Additionally, our study provides valuable insights into vascular access practices among populations living in under-resourced areas, who remain underrepresented in kidney health research despite being disproportionately affected by poor health outcomes. By examining data from a center specializing in hemodialysis (following the ISMMS model of care), this study contributes important evidence that may help inform future strategies to improve vascular access selection and patient outcomes in hemodialysis patients living in under-resourced areas.

5. Conclusions

In conclusion, this study underscores vascular access type as a key determinant of long-term survival in hemodialysis patients, with AVFs providing significant survival benefits over both tunneled and non-tunneled catheters. These findings reinforce the need to prioritize AVFs as the preferred vascular access, emphasizing the importance of early nephrology referral, patient education, and structural interventions to ensure timely AVF placement and maturation. This is particularly critical for older adults and diabetic patients, whose survival may heavily depend on having optimal vascular access. Addressing modifiable risk factors, such as diabetes management and infection prevention, is essential to improving vascular access outcomes in this high-risk population. Future research should focus on optimizing vascular access care, identifying barriers to AVF utilization, and developing strategies to enhance equitable access across diverse healthcare settings. Additionally, further studies are needed to evaluate the impact of multidisciplinary care models in improving vascular access planning and reducing disparities in access selection and outcomes.

Author Contributions: Conceptualization, I.D.-E.; data curation, A.F.-G.; formal analysis, J.V.-R., J.D.-M., R.T.-V., A.F.-G., J.G.-E., D.A.-F. and C.M.-R.; funding acquisition, I.D.-E.; investigation, J.V.-R., J.I.N.-C., P.C.-S., C.D. and A.C.E.-M.; methodology, J.V.-R., G.A.H.-F., C.S.P., J.D.-M., P.C.-S., C.D., R.T.-V., A.C.E.-M., D.A.-F. and I.D.-E.; project administration, I.D.-E.; resources, J.G.-E. and I.D.-E.; software, G.A.H.-F., A.C.E.-M., A.F.-G. and C.M.-R.; supervision, I.D.-E.; validation, C.S.P., J.I.N.-C., P.C.-S., R.T.-V. and I.D.-E.; visualization, I.D.-E.; writing—original draft, G.A.H.-F., J.D.-M. and I.D.-E.; writing—review and editing, G.A.H.-F. and I.D.-E. All authors have read and agreed to the published version of the manuscript.

Funding: This research received no external funding.

Institutional Review Board Statement: The study protocol was reviewed and approved by the local health research committee of IMSS-Colima, Mexico, under approval number R-2018-785-056 on 12 June 2018.

Informed Consent Statement: Informed consent was waived as the data were obtained retrospectively from clinical records and not directly from patients. All data were anonymized to protect patient confidentiality.

Data Availability Statement: The original contributions presented in the study are included in the article; further inquiries can be directed to the corresponding author.

Acknowledgments: The authors would like to thank Julio V. Barrios Nuñez from the ICEP Colima, Mexico, for their assistance with English language editing. G.A. Hernandez-Fuentes would like to express their gratitude for the financial support from SECIHTI, Mexico, for his postdoctoral studies (633738). The authors also extend their appreciation to the Health Research Security Institute for its support in conducting this research.

Conflicts of Interest: The authors declare no conflicts of interest.

References

1. Polanco-Flores, N.A. Chronic Renal Disease in Mexico: A Preventive Uncontrolled Epidemic. *Rev. Méd. Hosp. Gen. Méx.* **2019**, *82*, 194–197. [CrossRef]
2. Cueto-Manzano, A.M.; Rojas-Campos, E. Status of Renal Replacement Therapy and Peritoneal Dialysis in Mexico. *Perit. Dial. Int.* **2007**, *27*, 142–148. [CrossRef] [PubMed]
3. García-de-Alba-Verduzco, J.E.; García-de-Alba-Verduzco, J.E.; López-Elizalde, R.; García-de-Alba-García, J.E. Tabla de Vida Para Derechohabientes del Instituto de Seguridad y Servicios Sociales de Los Trabajadores Del Estado (ISSSTE), México 2021. *Cir. Cir.* **2024**, *92*, 594–602. [CrossRef] [PubMed]
4. Instituto Mexicano del Seguro Social (IMSS). Atiende IMSS a Cerca de 80 Mil Personas Con Terapia de Reemplazo Renal a Nivel Nacional. Available online: https://www.imss.gob.mx/prensa/archivo/202403/125 (accessed on 11 February 2025).
5. Saunders, H.; Rehan, A.; Hashmi, M.F.; Sanghavi, D.K. *Continuous Renal Replacement Therapy*; StatPearls Publishing: St. Petersburg, FL, USA, 2025.
6. Santoro, D.; Benedetto, F.; Mondello, P.; Pipitò, N.; Barillà, D.; Spinelli, F.; Ricciardi, C.A.; Cernaro, V.; Buemi, M. Vascular Access for Hemodialysis: Current Perspectives. *Int. J. Nephrol. Renovasc. Dis.* **2014**, *7*, 281–294. [CrossRef]
7. Lok, C.E.; Huber, T.S.; Orchanian-Cheff, A.; Rajan, D.K. Arteriovenous Access for Hemodialysis. *JAMA* **2024**, *331*, 1307–1317. [CrossRef]
8. García-Yañez, J.C.; Serrano-Gavuzzo, C.A.; Arvizu-Hernandez, M.; Moguel-González, B.; Bravo, E. Evaluation of Hemodialysis Vascular Access. Perspective from Mexico. *Front. Nephrol.* **2023**, *3*, 1084188. [CrossRef]
9. Lawson, J.H.; Niklason, L.E.; Roy-Chaudhury, P. Challenges and Novel Therapies for Vascular Access in Haemodialysis. *Nat. Rev. Nephrol.* **2020**, *16*, 586–602. [CrossRef]
10. Flick, A.I.; Winters, R. *Vascular Tunneled Central Catheter Access*; StatPearls Publishing: St. Petersburg, FL, USA, 2025.
11. Sohail, M.A.; Vachharajani, T.J.; Anvari, E. Central Venous Catheters for Hemodialysis—The Myth and the Evidence. *Kidney Int. Rep.* **2021**, *6*, 2958–2968. [CrossRef]
12. Murdeshwar, H.N.; Anjum, F. *Hemodialysis*; StatPearls Publishing: Treasure Island, FL, USA, 2025.
13. Pisoni, R.L.; Zepel, L.; Port, F.K.; Robinson, B.M. Trends in US Vascular Access Use, Patient Preferences, and Related Practices: An Update From the US DOPPS Practice Monitor With International Comparisons. *Am. J. Kidney Dis.* **2015**, *65*, 905–915. [CrossRef]
14. Pisoni, R.L.; Zepel, L.; Fluck, R.; Lok, C.E.; Kawanishi, H.; Süleymanlar, G.; Wasse, H.; Tentori, F.; Zee, J.; Li, Y.; et al. International Differences in the Location and Use of Arteriovenous Accesses Created for Hemodialysis: Results From the Dialysis Outcomes and Practice Patterns Study (DOPPS). *Am. J. Kidney Dis.* **2018**, *71*, 469–478. [CrossRef]
15. Contreras-Jimenez, E.; Lopez-Pena, G.; Ruben-Castillo, C.; Mier y Teran-Ellis, S.; Cuen-Ojeda, C.; Arzola-Flores, L.H.; Anaya-Ayala, J.E.; Hinojosa-Becerril, C.A. Análisis de Los Resultados Clínicos de Fístulas Arteriovenosas Para Acceso de Hemodiálisis En Población Adulta Mayor Mexicana. *Cir. Cir.* **2023**, *91*, 200–203. [CrossRef] [PubMed]
16. Patel, D.M.; Churilla, B.M.; Lee, T.C.; Thamer, M.; Zhang, Y.; Allon, M.; Crews, D.C. Patient Perspectives on Arteriovenous Fistula Placement, Maturation, and Use: A Qualitative Study. *Kidney Med.* **2024**, *6*, 100919. [CrossRef] [PubMed]
17. Murea, M.; Grey, C.R.; Lok, C.E. Shared Decision-Making in Hemodialysis Vascular Access Practice. *Kidney Int.* **2021**, *100*, 799–808. [CrossRef]

18. Jayroe, H.; Foley, K. *Arteriovenous Fistula*, 1st ed.; StatPearls Publishing: Treasure Island, FL, USA, 2025; Volume 1.
19. Tan, E.K.; Tan, S.G. The Permanent Catheter. *Hemodial. Int.* **2014**, *18*, 522–524. [CrossRef]
20. Clark, E.G.; Barsuk, J.H. Temporary Hemodialysis Catheters: Recent Advances. *Kidney Int.* **2014**, *86*, 888–895. [CrossRef]
21. World Medical Association. Declaration of Helsinki: Ethical Principles for Medical Research Involving Human Subjects. *JAMA* **2013**, *310*, 2191. [CrossRef]
22. Brown, R.S.; Patibandla, B.K.; Goldfarb-Rumyantzev, A.S. The Survival Benefit of "Fistula First, Catheter Last" in Hemodialysis Is Primarily Due to Patient Factors. *J. Am. Soc. Nephrol.* **2017**, *28*, 645–652. [CrossRef]
23. Rosner, B. *Fundamentals of Biostatistics*, 7th ed.; Cengage Learning, Inc.: Boston, MA, USA, 2010; Volume 1.
24. Andrade, C. Survival Analysis, Kaplan-Meier Curves, and Cox Regression: Basic Concepts. *Indian J. Psychol. Med.* **2023**, *45*, 434–435. [CrossRef]
25. Tolia, M.; Gkantaifi, A.; Hayward, L.; Gupta, G.; Kyriazoglou, A.; Mauri, D.; Nixon, I. Superficial Soft Tissue Sarcomas: 10-year Survival Outcomes. *Oncol. Lett.* **2023**, *25*, 96. [CrossRef]
26. Lundgreen, C.S.; Larson, D.R.; Atkinson, E.J.; Devick, K.L.; Lewallen, D.G.; Berry, D.J.; Maradit Kremers, H.; Crowson, C.S. Adjusted Survival Curves Improve Understanding of Multivariable Cox Model Results. *J. Arthroplast.* **2021**, *36*, 3367–3371. [CrossRef]
27. Post-Hoc Power Calculator Post-Hoc Power Calculator. Evaluate Statistical Power of an Existing Study. Available online: https://clincalc.com/stats/Power.aspx (accessed on 28 April 2023).
28. Mendoza-Hernandez, M.A.; Guzman-Esquivel, J.; Ramos-Rojas, M.A.; Santillan-Luna, V.V.; Sanchez-Ramirez, C.A.; Hernandez-Fuentes, G.A.; Diaz-Martinez, J.; Melnikov, V.; Rojas-Larios, F.; Martinez-Fierro, M.L.; et al. Differences in the Evolution of Clinical, Biochemical, and Hematological Indicators in Hospitalized Patients with COVID-19 According to Their Vaccination Scheme: A Cohort Study in One of the World's Highest Hospital Mortality Populations. *Vaccines* **2024**, *12*, 72. [CrossRef] [PubMed]
29. VanderWeele, T.J. On the Distinction Between Interaction and Effect Modification. *Epidemiology* **2009**, *20*, 863–871. [CrossRef]
30. Hart, J.E.; Puett, R.C.; Rexrode, K.M.; Albert, C.M.; Laden, F. Effect Modification of Long-Term Air Pollution Exposures and the Risk of Incident Cardiovascular Disease in US Women. *J. Am. Heart Assoc.* **2015**, *4*, e357. [CrossRef] [PubMed]
31. Diaz-Martinez, J.; Kotzker, W.; Mendoza-Hernandez, M.A.; Gadh, R.S.; Hernandez-Fuentes, G.A.; Bañuelos, A.; Guzmán-Esquivel, J.; Hong, A.; Delgado-Enciso, O.G.; Geyer-Roberts, E.; et al. Analysis of Survival Modification by Furosemide Use in a Cohort of Hospitalized COVID-19 Patients with Severe or Critical Disease in Mexico: Due to Its Chemical Structure, Furosemide Is More than Just a Diuretic. *Pharmaceutics* **2024**, *16*, 920. [CrossRef] [PubMed]
32. Allon, M. Vascular Access for Hemodialysis Patients. *Clin. J. Am. Soc. Nephrol.* **2019**, *14*, 954–961. [CrossRef]
33. Ahmadi, S.-F.; Streja, E.; Zahmatkesh, G.; Streja, D.; Kashyap, M.; Moradi, H.; Molnar, M.Z.; Reddy, U.; Amin, A.N.; Kovesdy, C.P.; et al. Reverse Epidemiology of Traditional Cardiovascular Risk Factors in the Geriatric Population. *J. Am. Med. Dir. Assoc.* **2015**, *16*, 933–939. [CrossRef]
34. Kovesdy, C.P.; Anderson, J.E. Cardiovascular and survival paradoxes in dialysis patients: Reverse epidemiology in patients with chronic kidney disease who are not yet on dialysis. *Semin. Dial.* **2007**, *20*, 566–569. [CrossRef]
35. Woodside, K.J.; Bell, S.; Mukhopadhyay, P.; Repeck, K.J.; Robinson, I.T.; Eckard, A.R.; Dasmunshi, S.; Plattner, B.W.; Pearson, J.; Schaubel, D.E.; et al. Arteriovenous Fistula Maturation in Prevalent Hemodialysis Patients in the United States: A National Study. *Am. J. Kidney Dis.* **2018**, *71*, 793–801. [CrossRef]
36. Levin, N.W.; Handelman, G.J.; Coresh, J.; Port, F.K.; Kaysen, G.A. Reverse Epidemiology: A Confusing, Confounding, and Inaccurate Term. *Semin. Dial.* **2007**, *20*, 586–592. [CrossRef]
37. Nlandu, Y.; Lepira, F.; Makulo, J.-R.; Engole, Y.; Sumaili, E.; Wameso, M.-N.; Mokoli, V.; Luse, J.; Longo, A.; Zinga, C.; et al. Reverse Epidemiology of Elevated Blood Pressure among Chronic Hemodialysis Black Patients with Stroke: A Historical Cohort Study. *BMC Nephrol.* **2017**, *18*, 277. [CrossRef]
38. Boulet, N.; Pensier, J.; Occean, B.-V.; Peray, P.F.; Mimoz, O.; Rickard, C.M.; Buetti, N.; Lefrant, J.-Y.; Muller, L.; Roger, C. Central Venous Catheter-Related Infections: A Systematic Review, Meta-Analysis, Trial Sequential Analysis and Meta-Regression Comparing Ultrasound Guidance and Landmark Technique for Insertion. *Crit. Care* **2024**, *28*, 378. [CrossRef] [PubMed]
39. Murea, M.; Geary, R.L.; Houston, D.K.; Edwards, M.S.; Robinson, T.W.; Davis, R.P.; Huric, J.B.; Williams, T.K.; Velazquez-Ramirez, G.; Bagwell, B.; et al. A Randomized Pilot Study to Evaluate Graft versus Fistula Vascular Access Strategy in Older Patients with Advanced Kidney Disease: Results of a Feasibility Study. *Pilot. Feasibility Stud.* **2020**, *6*, 86. [CrossRef] [PubMed]
40. Ikizler, T.A.; Burrowes, J.D.; Byham-Gray, L.D.; Campbell, K.L.; Carrero, J.-J.; Chan, W.; Fouque, D.; Friedman, A.N.; Ghaddar, S.; Goldstein-Fuchs, D.J.; et al. KDOQI Clinical Practice Guideline for Nutrition in CKD: 2020 Update. *Am. J. Kidney Dis.* **2020**, *76*, S1–S107. [CrossRef] [PubMed]
41. Sattar, A.; Argyropoulos, C.; Weissfeld, L.; Younas, N.; Fried, L.; Kellum, J.A.; Unruh, M. All-Cause and Cause-Specific Mortality Associated with Diabetes in Prevalent Hemodialysis Patients. *BMC Nephrol.* **2012**, *13*, 130. [CrossRef]
42. Zarkowsky, D.S.; Arhuidese, I.J.; Hicks, C.W.; Canner, J.K.; Qazi, U.; Obeid, T.; Schneider, E.; Abularrage, C.J.; Freischlag, J.A.; Malas, M.B. Racial/Ethnic Disparities Associated With Initial Hemodialysis Access. *JAMA Surg.* **2015**, *150*, 529. [CrossRef]

43. Griva, K.; Seow, P.S.; Seow, T.Y.-Y.; Goh, Z.S.; Choo, J.C.J.; Foo, M.; Newman, S. Patient-Related Barriers to Timely Dialysis Access Preparation: A Qualitative Study of the Perspectives of Patients, Family Members, and Health Care Providers. *Kidney Med.* **2020**, *2*, 29–41. [CrossRef]
44. Woo, K.; Pieters, H. The Patient Experience of Hemodialysis Vascular Access Decision-Making. *J. Vasc. Access* **2021**, *22*, 911–919. [CrossRef]
45. Mckeon, K.; Sibbel, S.; Brunelli, S.M.; Matheson, E.; Lefeber, N.; Epps, M.; Tentori, F. Utilization of Home Dialysis and Permanent Vascular Access at Dialysis Initiation Following a Structured CKD Education Program. *Kidney Med.* **2022**, *4*, 100490. [CrossRef]
46. MacRae, J.M.; Oliver, M.; Clark, E.; Dipchand, C.; Hiremath, S.; Kappel, J.; Kiaii, M.; Lok, C.; Luscombe, R.; Miller, L.M.; et al. Arteriovenous Vascular Access Selection and Evaluation. *Can. J. Kidney Health Dis.* **2016**, *3*, 2054358116669125. [CrossRef]
47. Fila, B.; Ibeas, J.; Tey, R.R.; Lovčić, V.; Zibar, L. Arteriovenous Fistula for Haemodialysis: The Role of Surgical Experience and Vascular Access Education. *Nefrología* **2016**, *36*, 89–94. [CrossRef]
48. Leblic Ramírez, I.; Riera del Moral, L.; Sánchez Villanueva, R.; Stefanov Kiuri, S.; Álvarez García, L.; Echarri Carrillo, R.; Gallegos Villalobos, Á.; Fernandez Heredero, Á. Effect of a Multidisciplinary Team in the Management of Vascular Access for Hemodialysis. *Nefrol. (Engl. Ed.)* **2024**, *44*, 450–452. [CrossRef] [PubMed]
49. Lee, W.; Campoy, S.; Smits, G.; Vu Tran, Z.; Chonchol, M. Effectiveness of a Chronic Kidney Disease Clinic in Achieving K/DOQI Guideline Targets at Initiation of Dialysis--a Single-Centre Experience. *Nephrol. Dial. Transplant.* **2007**, *22*, 833–838. [CrossRef] [PubMed]
50. Wei, S.; Chang, Y.; Mau, L.; Lin, M.; Chiu, H.; Tsai, J.; Huang, C.; Chen, H.; HWANG, S. Chronic Kidney Disease Care Program Improves Quality of Pre-end-stage Renal Disease Care and Reduces Medical Costs. *Nephrology* **2010**, *15*, 108–115. [CrossRef] [PubMed]
51. Yeoh, H.H.; Tiquia, H.S.; Abcar, A.C.; Rasgon, S.A.; Idroos, M.L.; Daneshvari, S.F. Impact of Predialysis Care on Clinical Outcomes. *Hemodial. Int.* **2003**, *7*, 338–341. [CrossRef]
52. Levin, A.; Lewis, M.; Mortiboy, P.; Faber, S.; Hare, I.; Porter, E.C.; Mendelssohn, D.C. Multidisciplinary Predialysis Programs: Quantification and Limitations of Their Impact on Patient Outcomes in Two Canadian Settings. *Am. J. Kidney Dis.* **1997**, *29*, 533–540. [CrossRef]
53. Elliott, M.J.; Ravani, P.; Quinn, R.R.; Oliver, M.J.; Love, S.; MacRae, J.; Hiremath, S.; Friesen, S.; James, M.T.; King-Shier, K.M. Patient and Clinician Perspectives on Shared Decision Making in Vascular Access Selection: A Qualitative Study. *Am. J. Kidney Dis.* **2023**, *81*, 48–58.e1. [CrossRef]
54. Wong, T.-S.; Chen, Q.; Liu, T.; Yu, J.; Gao, Y.; He, Y.; Zhong, Q.; Tan, Z.; Liu, T.; Lu, J.; et al. Patients, Healthcare Providers, and General Population Preferences for Hemodialysis Vascular Access: A Discrete Choice Experiment. *Front. Public Health* **2024**, *12*, 1047769. [CrossRef]
55. Bikbov, B.; Purcell, C.A.; Levey, A.S.; Smith, M.; Abdoli, A.; Abebe, M.; Adebayo, O.M.; Afarideh, M.; Agarwal, S.K.; Agudelo-Botero, M.; et al. Global, Regional, and National Burden of Chronic Kidney Disease, 1990–2017: A Systematic Analysis for the Global Burden of Disease Study 2017. *Lancet* **2020**, *395*, 709–733. [CrossRef]
56. Méndez-Durán, A. Evolución Del Tratamiento Sustitutivo de La Función Renal En México En Los Últimos 10 Años. *Nefrología* **2021**, *41*, 82–83. [CrossRef]

medicina

MDPI

Article

Serum Endocan as a Predictor of Survival and Cardiovascular Events in Patients Without Diabetic Kidney Disease on Chronic Haemodialysis: A Prospective, Observational Study

Mario Šafer [1,2], Ivan Feldi [2,3], Ines Šahinović [2,4], Ivana Tolj [2,5], Marko Pirić [2,6], Dunja Šojat [2,6], Eduard Oštarijaš [7,*] and Dubravka Mihaljević [2,5]

1 Department of Internal Medicine, General Hospital Virovitica, Lj. Gaja 21, 33000 Virovitica, Croatia; mario.safer27@gmail.com
2 Faculty of Medicine Osijek, Josip Juraj Strossmayer University of Osijek, J. Huttlera 4, 31000 Osijek, Croatia; ivanatolj5@gmail.com (I.T.)
3 Department of Internal Medicine, General County Hospital Našice, 31500 Našice, Croatia
4 Clinical Institute for Laboratory Diagnostics, Clinical Hospital Centre Osijek, J. Huttlera 4, 31000 Osijek, Croatia
5 Department of Nephrology, Clinic of Internal Medicine, Clinical Hospital Centre Osijek, J. Huttlera 4, 31000 Osijek, Croatia
6 Health Centre of Osijek-Baranja County, Park Kralja Petra Krešimira IV. 6, 31000 Osijek, Croatia
7 Doctoral School of Clinical Medical Sciences, Medical School, University of Pécs, Szigeti út 12, 7624 Pécs, Hungary
* Correspondence: eduard.ostarijas@aok.pte.hu

Abstract: *Background and Objectives*: Chronic kidney disease (CKD) is an increasingly significant global public health issue, with cardiovascular disease being the leading cause of mortality. Endothelial dysfunction plays a critical role, but diagnostic tools have certain limitations. Endocan, a soluble proteoglycan, emerged as a promising endothelial dysfunction marker and potential major adverse cardiovascular event (MACE) predictor in haemodialysis (HD) patients. *Materials and Methods*: In this single-centre, observational, prospective study, non-diabetic HD patients without prior MACEs were monitored. A total of 75 participants met the inclusion criteria. We measured serum endocan, standard biochemical and anthropometric parameters, and parameters of peripheral and central haemodynamics before and after HD in all participants. *Results*: Patients with higher endocan were older, had elevated CRP and reduced albumin concentrations, and often had a tunnelled central venous catheter (TCVC) for vascular access. Higher serum endocan levels were independently associated with an increased risk of MACEs (aHR = 4.09, 95%-CI: 1.72–9.74), MACE-related mortality (aHR = 2.64, 95%-CI: 1.23–5.66), and all-cause mortality (aHR = 1.86, 95%-CI: 1.07–3.23), both before and after adjusting for predefined confounders, with the highest endocan tercile exhibiting the shortest event-free survival. *Conclusions*: Endocan is a valuable marker of inflammation and endothelial dysfunction in non-diabetic HD patients. Its elevated concentration indicates an increased cardiovascular risk and more frequent MACEs. Future multicentre studies with repeated endocan assessments should validate its prognostic and diagnostic utility, particularly in long-term patient follow-up.

Keywords: endothelial dysfunction; haemodialysis; endocan; MACE

1. Introduction

Chronic kidney disease (CKD) is a growing global public health concern, with a prevalence of approximately 8% to 16% [1]. Cardiovascular disease (CVD) is the primary cause of morbidity and mortality in both CKD and end-stage kidney disease (ESKD) [2,3]. Approximately, 2 out of 1000 patients with CKD (0.2%) have ESKD and are on dialysis [4]. Mortality among individuals on dialysis is high, and sudden cardiac arrest (SCA) accounts for a large percentage, with estimates ranging from 14% to 45% [5–7]. In patients undergoing dialysis, SCA events were significantly more common on dialysis days and 3-fold higher than expected by chance [8]. Diabetic kidney disease is the leading cause of ESKD, accounting for 30% to 50% of the incident cases in the United States and most developed countries [9], but diabetes itself is also an independent risk factor for CKD progression and CVD. Among various traditional and non-traditional risk factors linking CKD and CVD, endothelial dysfunction stands out as a key contributor, which manifests as endothelial cell activation leading to vasoconstriction, inflammation, and a pro-atherothrombotic state [10,11]. Current methods of assessing endothelial dysfunction—ranging from invasive coronary flow measurements to non-invasive flow-mediated dilation (FMD)—have limitations due to invasiveness, high costs, and technical demand [12]. Hence, there is a need for novel biomarkers of endothelial dysfunction.

Endocan, a proteoglycan secreted by activated endothelial cells, has emerged as a promising marker of endothelial dysfunction. It is involved in regulating cell adhesion, migration, proliferation, and neovascularisation, and it has shown promising utility in various kidney disease entities, including ESKD [13–19]. Higher endocan levels have been associated with major endothelial damage, the progression of CKD, an increased likelihood of transplant rejection, and higher rates of cardiovascular events (CVEs) and mortality [20,21]. Although previous studies have investigated the role of endocan in this context, its role specifically in patients without diabetes but with CKD remains less explored.

In this study, we specifically measured serum levels of endocan and parameters of central and peripheral haemodynamics in non-diabetic HD patients without prior major adverse cardiovascular events (MACEs) to investigate its potential as a marker of vascular dysfunction independent of diabetes. Additionally, the study examined how endocan is linked to MACEs and multiple survival parameters over the follow-up period. A MACE is a composite clinical endpoint including myocardial infarction, stroke, hospitalisation for heart failure, and cardiovascular death.

2. Materials and Methods

2.1. Study Population and Design

This is a single-centre, non-randomised, observational, prospective cohort study that was conducted from March 2018 until March 2023 at the Department of Nephrology, Clinical Hospital Centre Osijek, Croatia. A total of 75 patients of both genders who met the inclusion criteria were included in the research. The inclusion criteria were as follows: the participants were older than 18 years, had been on haemodialysis for at least 3 months, were dialysed 3 times a week for 4 h using the haemodiafiltration modality, and had to be anuric with a maximum urine output of up to 200 mL in 24 h. Also, their Kt/V, as a measure of dialysis adequacy, had to be >1.4. Patients were excluded if they were undergoing active oncologic treatment or if less than five years had passed since the completion of cancer therapy; if they had atrial fibrillation with rapid ventricular response accompanied by symptomatic heart failure at the time of enrolment; if they had undergone lower limb amputation; if they had active symptoms or a confirmed and treated systemic inflammatory or infectious disease at the time of enrolment; if they had diabetes mellitus; or if they had a history of MACEs. A MACE was defined as acute coronary syndrome, cerebrovascular insult, or hospitalisation due to an episode of acute heart failure. Each patient was informed about all protocols and procedures of this research, and all participants signed an informed consent form for participation, which adhered to all modern ethical and deontological principles. The study protocol adhered to the standards established by the latest revision of the Declaration of Helsinki and was approved by the Ethics Committee of the Faculty of Medicine Osijek and the Ethics Committee of the University Hospital Osijek (Number: R2-6782/2018, date of approval 3 May 2018). The study was conducted at the Department of Nephrology and the Clinical Institute for Laboratory Diagnostics, University Hospital Osijek.

2.2. Demographic Data, Anthropometric Analyses, and Biochemical Investigations

We analysed routine biochemical parameters, such as complete blood count, C-reactive protein (CRP), total cholesterol, low-density lipoprotein (LDL) cholesterol, glucose, albumin, calcium, phosphorus, parathyroid hormone (PTH), ferritin, and iron. These parameters were measured using standard methods. Plasma samples were collected using tubes treated with ethylenediaminetetraacetic acid (EDTA) on the day of enrolment in the study. Following centrifugation for 15 min at $1000\times g$ at room temperature, the samples were stored at -80 °C until analysis. A separate blood sample for serum analysis of endocan was obtained using commercially available enzyme-linked immunosorbent assay (ELISA) kits (using Magnetic Luminex® Screening Assay multiplex kits, R&D Systems, Minneapolis, MN, USA) at the Clinical Institute for Laboratory Diagnostics, Clinical Hospital Centre Osijek, Croatia.

Blood samples for biochemical analysis were obtained just before a midweek HD session (Wednesday or Thursday) together with measurements of parameters of central and peripheral haemodynamics. Hydration status is most stable before midweek sessions (e.g., Wednesday or Thursday), reducing variability due to fluid overload or excessive dehydration. Blood pressure and vascular tone are more consistent compared to post-dialysis, when vasodilation and volume shifts occur. Also, reproducibility is highest in this pre-dialysis, midweek window, making it the preferred standard.

Each participant was weighed before HD, and the total interdialytic weight gain (IWG) was recorded in relation to the estimated dry weight, which was assessed using the bioimpedance method with a body composition monitor (BCM) device (BCM, Fresenius Medical Care, Bad Homburg, Germany). Demographic data and medical history were obtained from the medical records of each participant. Accordingly, their age, gender, HD vintage, vascular access, aetiology of CKD, history of MACEs, malignant disease, inflammatory diseases, and diabetes were recorded.

MACEs, cardiovascular mortality, and all-cause mortality were the investigated outcomes. The cause of mortality was assessed from medical records and through interviews with attending physicians and family members. Participants who underwent kidney transplantation during the follow-up period were excluded from the study.

2.3. Assessments of Peripheral and Central Haemodynamic Parameters

Two consecutive measurements of pulse wave velocity (PWV), peripheral systolic and diastolic blood pressure (SBP and DBP), central aortic SBP and DBP, heart rate (HR), mean arterial pressure (MAP), pulse pressure (PP), and augmentation index (AI) were performed using a Mobil-O-Graph Agedio B900 device (IEM GmbH, Aachen, Germany) before and after a midweek HD session. The rationale for this was that immediately after dialysis, blood pressure drops, vessels dilate, and arterial stiffness can be underestimated, whereas the day after a long dialysis break, patients are often fluid overloaded, which can falsely increase arterial stiffness.

This non-invasive oscillometric device utilises integrated ARCSolver algorithms (Austrian Institute of Technology, Vienna, Austria) to derive aortic stiffness surrogates based on brachial blood pressure readings through a generalised transfer function. Measurements were performed in the supine position after 5 min of rest, using cuffs adapted to the circumference of the non-fistula arm. Blood samples for biochemical analysis were then obtained, and patients began their HD session. After 4 h of HD and a 5 min rest in the supine position, measurements were repeated following the same protocol.

2.4. Statistical Analysis

We summarised demographic, biochemical, and clinical characteristics across serum endocan levels stratified by terciles using descriptive statistics, with categorical variables compared using the chi-square test with continuity correction, normally distributed continuous variables using one-way ANOVA, and non-normally distributed continuous variables using the Kruskal–Wallis test. Count data were presented as a whole number (percentage), and normally distributed variables were presented as the mean ± standard deviation (SD), whereas non-normally distributed variables were expressed as the median [Q1, Q3]. The association of serum endocan levels with MACEs and mortality was assessed by a time-to-event analysis using Kaplan–Meier survival curves and Cox proportional hazards multivariate models, with serum endocan levels analysed both as a continuous variable and stratified into terciles. Hazard ratios (HRs) with 95% confidence intervals (95%-CI) were reported from the multivariable Cox models, adjusted for the predefined potential confounders selected based on clinical expertise: age, sex, HD vintage, albumin, BMI, central SBP, and AI. All analyses were performed in R version 4.4.1 (R Core Team, Vienna, Austria).

3. Results

3.1. Demographic, Clinical, and Biochemical Characteristics

The patients were enrolled in the study between March 2018 and March 2019 and were followed until March 2023. The median follow-up period was 40 [18.5, 60] months. During this time, a total of 156 patients were initially screened for eligibility. Following the exclusion of individuals who either did not meet the inclusion criteria or declined participation, 80 patients were ultimately enrolled for analysis and follow-up. A total of five patients received a kidney transplant during follow-up and were, therefore, excluded from further analyses. A flow diagram outlining the participant selection process is presented in Figure 1.

A total of 75 participants were included in the study and stratified into terciles based on serum endocan concentrations. Of these, 31 (41.3%) were women. The overall median age was 70 [59, 76.5] years, the median dialysis vintage was 52 months [21.5, 108.5], and there were 34 patients (45.33%) with a tunnelled central venous catheter (TCVC) for vascular access. Other, detailed baseline demographic, biochemical, and clinical characteristics of the study population, stratified by serum endocan concentrations, are reported in Table 1. Patients with higher levels of endocan were older (50.00 [41.00, 64.00], 71.00 [64.00, 75.00], and 77.00 [72.00, 81.00] years for first, second, and third terciles, respectively) and more frequently had a TCVC. The TCVC was significantly lower only in the first tercile, where there was a significantly higher number of patients with arteriovenous fistulas (AVFs). Other indicators such as gender, HD vintage, IWG, dialysis dose, aetiology of CKD, and the use of antihypertensive and hypolipemic medications were not statistically significantly associated with endocan levels.

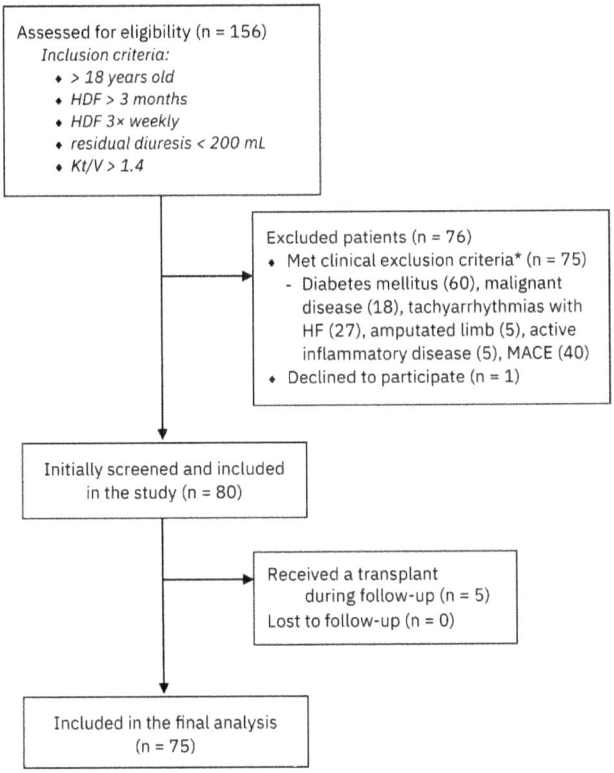

Figure 1. Participant selection process. HDF: haemodiafiltration; MACE: major adverse cardiovascular event. Note: * The sum of individual exclusion criteria exceeds the total number of excluded patients, as some patients fulfilled multiple exclusion criteria simultaneously.

Table 1. Demographic, clinical, and biochemical variables.

Parameters	1st Tercile of Serum Endocan Levels (2.99–4.67 μg/L)	2nd Tercile of Serum Endocan Levels (4.68–6.29 μg/L)	3rd Tercile of Serum Endocan Levels (6.30–7.93 μg/L)	*p*-Value
Number of patients	25 (33.3%)	25 (33.3%)	25 (33.3%)	
Sex				0.214
Male	18 (72.0)	14 (56.0)	12 (48.0)	
Female	7 (28.0)	11 (44.0)	13 (52.0)	
Age (years)	50.00 [41.00, 64.00]	71.00 [64.00, 75.00]	77.00 [72.00, 81.00]	<0.001
HD vintage (months)	31.00 [6.00, 96.00]	53.00 [21.00, 109.00]	62.00 [48.00, 97.00]	0.083
Interdialytic weight gain (kg)	2.56 (1.06)	2.28 (0.99)	2.44 (1.03)	0.629
Body mass index (kg/m^2)	27.39 [24.40, 30.44]	25.91 [22.50, 28.22]	26.40 [23.20, 29,70]	0.448
Diabetes mellitus	0 (0.0)	0 (0.0)	0 (0.0)	1.000

Table 1. *Cont.*

Parameters	1st Tercile of Serum Endocan Levels (2.99–4.67 μg/L)	2nd Tercile of Serum Endocan Levels (4.68–6.29 μg/L)	3rd Tercile of Serum Endocan Levels (6.30–7.93 μg/L)	*p*-Value
Vascular access				0.027
Central venous catheter	6 (24.0)	15 (60.0)	13 (52.0)	
AV fistula	19 (76.0)	10 (40.0)	12 (48.0)	
Follow up (months)	60.00 [60.00, 60.00]	38.00 [20.00, 60.00]	23.00 [14.00, 32.00]	<0.001
Dialysis dose (Kt/V)	1.61 (0.19)	1.66 (0.18)	1.67 (0.20)	0.491
Haematological counts				
Leucocytes (WBCs) ($\times 10^9$/L)	7.00 (1.86)	6.75 (2.08)	7.34 (2.25)	0.596
Erythrocytes (RBCs) ($\times 10^{12}$/L)	3.78 (0.46)	3.68 (0.43)	3.60 (0.43)	0.342
Haemoglobin concentration (g/L)	109.64 (10.24)	105.88 (9.50)	106.64 (8.26)	0.330
HbA1c (%)	4.8 [4.6, 5.1]	4.8 [4.5, 4.9]	4.9 [4.4, 5.0]	0.598
Thrombocytes ($\times 10^9$/L)	214.00 [178.00, 238.00]	189.00 [177.00, 275.00]	174.00 [135.00, 226.00]	0.369
Serum biochemical parameters				
CRP (mg/dL)	5.50 [4.50, 8.00]	7.80 [4.00, 13.42]	17.60 [11.80, 24.40]	<0.001
Albumin (g/L)	39.00 [36.70, 40.30]	36.60 [34.30, 37.90]	37.10 [35.20, 39.00]	0.026
Glucose (mmol/L)	4.80 [4.40, 5.10]	4.50 [4.30, 4.90]	4.70 [4.40, 5.00]	0.475
Iron (mmol/L)	10.20 [9.30, 12.10]	9.30 [7.60, 14.20]	8.90 [6.50, 11.10]	0.091
Ferritin (ng/mL)	289.00 [123.40, 437.50]	437.60 [252.70, 687.60]	434.90 [286.80, 546.00]	0.070
Total cholesterol (mmol/L)	4.53 (1.13)	4.43 (1.13)	3.96 (1.26)	0.196
LDL cholesterol (mmol/L)	2.12 [1.89, 2.67]	2.12 [1.76, 2.35]	1.87 [1.43, 2.23]	0.236
Calcium (mmol/L)	2.23 [2.07, 2.34]	2.33 [2.18, 2,41]	2.21 [2.04, 2.30]	0.139
Phosphorus (mmol/L)	1.77 (0.37)	1.63 (0.45)	1.58 (0.39)	0.491
PTH (pg/mL)	222.00 [112.00, 307.00]	348.00 [253.00, 423.00]	283.00 [162.00, 403.00]	0.085
Endocan (μg/L)	4.34 (0.47)	5.73 (0.36)	6.79 (0.40)	<0.001
Therapy:				
RAAS inhibitor (%)	15 (60.0)	19 (76.0)	15 (60.0)	0.390
Calcium channel blocker (%)	16 (64.0)	11 (44.0)	15 (60.0)	0.321
Beta blocker (%)	16 (64.0)	15 (60.0)	12 (48.0)	0.492
Statin (%)	15 (60.0)	17 (68.0)	15 (60.0)	0.796
Cause of ESKD:				0.447
Glomerulonephritis (%)	7 (28.0)	6 (24.0)	8 (32.0)	
Arterial hypertension (%)	5 (20.0)	7 (28.0)	9 (36.0)	
Chronic pyelonephritis (%)	3 (12.0)	4 (16.0)	3 (12.0)	
Polycystic kidney disease (%)	4 (16.0)	2 (8.0)	0 (0.0)	
Tubulointerstitial nephritis (%)	0 (0.0)	3 (12.0)	2 (8.0)	

HD: haemodialysis, AV: arteriovenous fistula, WBCs: white blood cells; RBCs: red blood cells; CRP: C-reactive protein, PTH: parathyroid hormone, RAAS: renin angiotensin aldosterone system, and ESKD: end-stage renal disease.

Regarding biochemical parameters, patients with higher endocan levels had significantly higher levels of CRP and lower serum albumin concentrations. Statistical significance for CRP was found between the first and third terciles, as well as between the second and third terciles. Statistical significance for albumin was noted only between the first and second terciles. The numbers of leukocytes, erythrocytes, platelets, haemoglobin, iron, ferritin, calcium, phosphorus, PTH, total cholesterol, and LDL cholesterol were not statistically associated with different serum endocan concentrations. A detailed analysis of all investigated variables can be found in Table 1, along with the notation of statistical significance.

3.2. Parameters of Peripheral and Central Haemodynamics

Peripheral and central haemodynamic parameters of the study population, according to serum endocan concentration, are summarised in Table 2. In the measurements taken before HD, higher values according to terciles were observed for peripheral SBP, MAP, PP, central aortic SBP, and central PP, with statistically significant differences found between the first and third terciles. For the AI, statistical significance was noted between the second and third terciles, as well as between the first and third terciles, while PWV was statistically significantly elevated across all terciles. In measurements taken after HD, both PWV and the AI retained statistical significance between all terciles. There were no statistically significant differences among the other parameters. A detailed analysis of all investigated variables can be found in Table 2, along with the notation of statistical significance.

Table 2. Parameters of peripheral and central haemodynamics.

Parameters	1st Tercile of Serum Endocan Levels (2.99–4.67 μg/L)	2nd Tercile of Serum Endocan Levels (4.68–6.29 μg/L)	3rd Tercile of Serum Endocan Levels (6.30–7.93 μg/L)	*p*-Value
PWV (m/s)	8.17 (1.22)	10.46 (1.64)	12.62 (1.51)	<0.001
PWV after HD (m/s)	7.88 (1.57)	10.36 (1.64)	11.94 (1.45)	<0.001
Peripheral SBP (mmHg)	143.00 [137.00, 152.00]	152.00 [125.00, 164.00]	157.00 [149.00, 173.00]	0.026
Peripheral DBP (mmHg)	88.20 (14.07)	87.36 (14.98)	93.28 (14.83)	0.308
MAP (mmHg)	112.00 [98.00, 122.00]	117.00 [100.00, 121.00]	120.00 [114.00, 134.00]	0.049
PP (mmHg)	55.40 (8.09)	62.64 (19.62)	69.88 (19.59)	0.012
HR (per minute)	75.00 [72.00, 79.00]	71.13 [64.00, 74.00]	70.00 [60.00, 78.00]	0.151
AI	23.48 (8.23)	27.36 (15.05)	38.56 (10.38)	<0.001
Central SBP (mmHg)	130.00 [126.00, 141.00]	133.00 [118.00, 148.00]	146.00 [131.00, 163.00]	0.024
Central DBP (mmHg)	88.12 (15.57)	87.64 (15.58)	94.60 (15.24)	0.213
Central PP (mmHg)	43.00 [39.00, 47.00]	46.00 [38.00, 49.00]	51.00 [44.00, 69.00]	0.029
Peripheral SBP after HD (mmHg)	130.00 [120.00, 140.00]	142.00 [125.00, 162.00]	149.00 [131.00, 158.00]	0.059
Peripheral DBP after HD (mmHg)	84.16 (14.82)	84.60 (19.17)	86.24 (14.97)	0.895
MAP after HD (mmHg)	100.00 [92.00, 116.00]	104.00 [96.00, 127.00]	117.00 [104.00, 125.00]	0.143
PP after HD (mmHg)	52.00 [41.00, 58.00]	58.00 [47.00, 67.00]	61.00 [48.00, 73.00]	0.124
HR after HD (per minute)	83.52 (14.41)	77.91 (11.52)	75.47 (12.79)	0.087
AI after HD	18.00 [13.00, 32.00]	30.00 [15.00, 40.00]	30.00 [19.00, 43.00]	0.036
Central SBP after HD (mmHg)	124.64 (17.96)	131.88 (22.78)	133.60 (19.55)	0.257
Central DBP after HD (mmHg)	84.64 (16.58)	85.20 (20.22)	88.20 (14.80)	0.738
Central PP after HD (mmHg)	42.00 [30.00, 50.00]	47.00 [34.00, 55.00]	44.00 [33.00, 53.00]	0.461

PWV: pulse wave velocity, SBP: systolic blood pressure, DBP: diastolic blood pressure, MAP: mean arterial pressure, PP: pulse pressure, HR: heart rate, and AI: augmentation index.

3.3. Outcomes and Survival

The total average follow-up period was 40 months [18.5, 60]. During the follow-up period, a total of 32 MACEs were recorded, of which 20 out of 32 (62.5%) occurred in the third tercile of serum endocan levels, which was statistically significant. Of the total number of patients who started the study, 46 out of 75 (61.33%) died; 29 out of 46 (63.04%) died from MACEs, while 17 out of 46 (36.96%) died from other causes. Among the survivors, 21 out of 29 (72.41%) were in the first tercile of serum endocan levels, while 20 out of 29 (68.97%) of those who died from MACEs were in the third tercile, which was statistically significant. A detailed analysis of all investigated variables can be found in Table 3, along with the notation of statistical significance.

Table 3. Association between serum endocan levels and observed outcomes.

Parameters	1st Tercile of Serum Endocan Levels (2.99–4.67 μg/L)	2nd Tercile of Serum Endocan Levels (4.68–6.29 μg/L)	3rd Tercile of Serum Endocan Levels (6.30–7.93 μg/L)	*p*-Value
Number of patients	25 (33.3)	25 (33.3)	25 (33.3)	
Number of patients who experienced a major adverse cardiovascular event (MACE) (%)	3 (12.0)	9 (36.0)	20 (80.0)	<0.001
Cause of death:				<0.001
not applicable (surviving participants) (%)	21 (84.0)	8 (32.0)	0 (0.0)	
MACE (%)	1 (4.0)	8 (32.0)	20 (80.0)	
other causes (%)	3 (12.0)	9 (36.0)	5 (20.0)	

Time-to-event analysis using Kaplan–Meier survival curves and Cox proportional hazards multivariate models adjusted for the predefined potential confounders (i.e., age, sex, HD vintage, albumin, BMI, central SBP, and AI) are reported in Figure 2. One initially preselected variable (pulse wave velocity) was excluded from the final multivariate model due to a very strong collinearity with serum endocan levels (Spearman's rho = 0.82, $p < 0.0001$) in order to not compromise model stability and interpretability. Higher serum endocan levels were independently associated with an increased incidence of MACEs (aHR = 4.09, 95%-CI: 1.72–9.74, $p = 0.0014$), MACE-related mortality (aHR = 2.64, 95%-CI: 1.23–5.66, $p = 0.012$), and increased all-cause mortality (aHR = 1.86, 95%-CI: 1.07–3.23, $p = 0.027$), both before and after adjusting for predefined confounders, with the highest endocan tercile exhibiting the shortest event-free survival. Detailed model results with all variables are displayed in Table 4. To assess the robustness of the association, we additionally utilised a reduced model constructed via stepwise variable selection based on univariate significance ($p < 0.05$), in which endocan levels remained statistically significant.

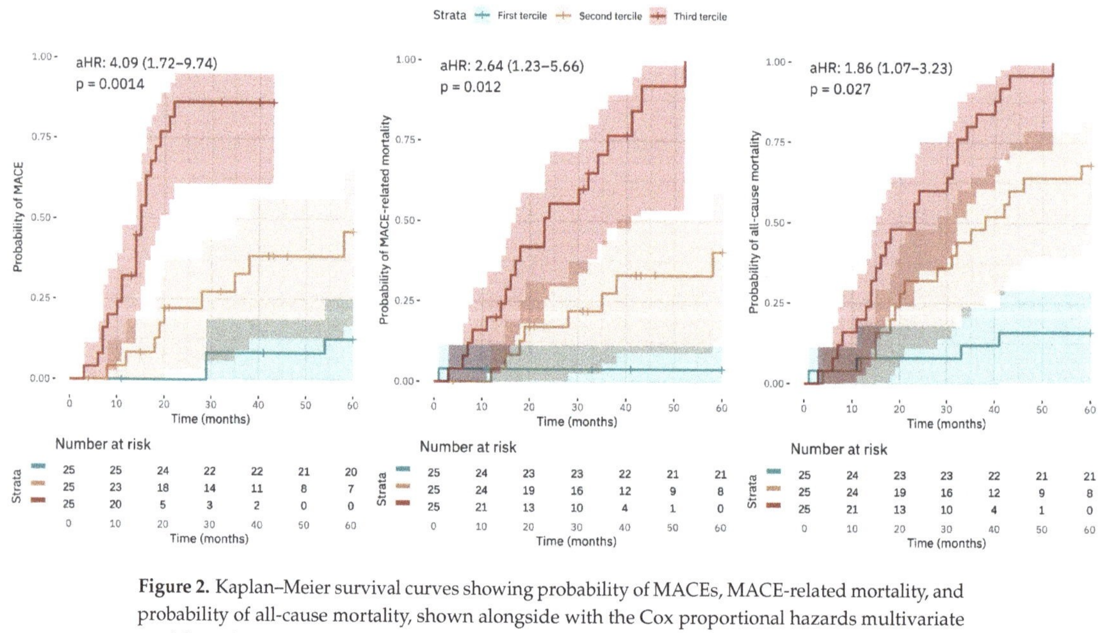

Figure 2. Kaplan–Meier survival curves showing probability of MACEs, MACE-related mortality, and probability of all-cause mortality, shown alongside with the Cox proportional hazards multivariate model results.

Table 4. Detailed results of the Cox multivariate model.

Outcome	MACE		MACE-Related Mortality		All-Cause Mortality	
Variable	HR (95%-CI)	p-Value	HR (95%-CI)	p-Value	HR (95%-CI)	p-Value
Serum endocan concentration	4.09 (1.72–9.74)	0.00144	2.64 (1.23–5.65)	0.0125	1.86 (1.07–3.23)	0.0272
Age	1.01 (0.96–1.07)	0.711	1.02 (0.97–1.08)	0.386	1.03 (0.99–1.08)	0.11
Sex (male)	1.96 (0.87–4.41)	0.103	1.04 (0.46–2.37)	0.921	1.30 (0.67–2.52)	0.434
Duration of haemodialysis	1.01 (1.00–1.01)	0.0688	1.00 (1.00–1.01)	0.284	1.01 (1.00–1.01)	0.00778
Serum albumin concentration	0.98 (0.85–1.12)	0.736	1.05 (0.91–1.22)	0.504	0.99 (0.89–1.10)	0.824
BMI	1.00 (0.93–1.07)	0.997	0.99 (0.92–1.06)	0.751	0.99 (0.93–1.05)	0.638
Central systolic pressure	0.99 (0.98–1.01)	0.453	1.00 (0.99–1.02)	0.731	1.00 (0.99–1.02)	0.48
Augmentation index	1.01 (0.98–1.04)	0.7	1.02 (0.99–1.05)	0.253	1.00 (0.98–1.03)	0.926

MACE: major adverse cardiovascular event, HR: hazard ratio, and BMI: body mass index.

4. Discussion

Our main findings are that patients with higher serum endocan levels had an increased risk of MACEs, MACE-related mortality, and all-cause mortality, both before and after adjusting for predefined confounders, with the highest endocan tercile exhibiting the shortest event-free survival in the population of patients without DKD and prior MACEs.

Our study is distinguished from previous research by the exclusion of patients with DKD and those with a history of MACEs prior to enrolment; such an approach ensured a unique study population. Given that earlier studies have demonstrated the substantial impact of diabetes and prior MACEs on endocan concentrations and future cardiovascular outcomes, our results further reinforce the significance of endocan as a potential biomarker that can be used as an independent cardiovascular risk factor in HD patients.

Other studies have also investigated the impact of endocan on the occurrence of MACEs and survival in populations of patients with CKD, those on HD, and those on PD. Several studies in CKD and PD populations demonstrated that serum endocan is associated with survival and both fatal and non-fatal MACEs [17,22]. In a population of patients on HD, Kim et al. evaluated the potential predictive role of endocan for cardiovascular risk in HD patients. The high-endocan group experienced more frequent MACEs, and endocan served as an independent predictor of MACEs in patients on HD [23]. Lin et al. established a correlation between higher endocan levels and all-cause mortality in HD patients [24]. Wu et al. concluded that among patients on maintenance HD, serum endocan levels positively correlated with the surrogate marker of aortic stiffness, both in a dose-dependent manner and with significant predictive power [25]. It is important to reiterate that the studies conducted by Kim et al., Wu et al., and Lin et al. included participants with diabetes and those with a prior history of MACEs, both of which are independent risk factors for (subsequent) MACEs.

In CKD, traditional risk factors cannot explain the high prevalence of CVD disease [26]. Factors related to endothelial dysfunction have increasingly been studied [21]. Several studies have demonstrated that endocan is involved in endothelial dysfunction and inflammation and could be an independent risk factor for poor clinical outcomes in CVD and CKD [23,27–29].

We showed that patients with higher serum concentrations of endocan were older, had higher levels of CRP, and lower albumin levels. It is expected that arteries will be stiffer and that endothelial dysfunction will be more pronounced with aging. Persistent inflammation results in a lower albumin concentration and leads to the deterioration of endothelial dysfunction. Statistically significant declines in albumin levels begin in the second tercile of endocan concentration, suggesting that patients enter a catabolic phase and a state of chronic inflammation relatively quickly. Similar findings were reported by other authors, albeit in populations of CKD patients who were not yet on HD and in patients on PD. For instance, Yilmaz et al. studied plasma endocan levels in non-dialysed CKD patients at stages 1–5 (n = 215) in relation to inflammation, endothelial dysfunction, MACE incidence, and overall survival. They found that plasma endocan concentration correlated with the estimated glomerular filtration rate, different markers of inflammation (pentraxin 3 and high-sensitivity CRP (hs-CRP), FMV, and carotid intima–media thickness (CIMT) [22]. Pawlak et al. conducted a cross-sectional study in non-dialysed CKD patients (n = 53) with and without CVD, aiming to evaluate plasma endocan, soluble intercellular adhesion molecule-1 (sICAM-1), soluble vascular adhesion molecule-1 (sVCAM-1), markers of inflammation (hs-CRP, interleukin-6, and tumour necrosis factor-α), and their inter-relations. They found that plasma endocan, sICAM-1, sVCAM-1, and hs-CRP levels were significantly higher in CKD patients than in controls and also significantly higher in CKD patients with CVD than in those without CVD [29]. Poon et al. examined the relationship between serum endocan level and clinical outcomes of PD patients (n = 193). The results revealed that patients with higher serum endocan levels in tercile 3 had lower serum albumin levels, higher carotid–femoral PWV, and higher CRP than those in terciles 2 and 1. Similar to our findings, they observed a close correlation between serum endocan and CRP levels, suggesting that endocan may be involved in systemic inflammation, a notion supported by the recent literature indicating that it partly modulates leukocyte diapedesis [17,22,23].

In the group of patients with higher endocan, we observed that TCVCs were more frequently used for vascular access to HD. Statistically, this was significant for the first tercile, where AVFs dominated. We hypothesise that patients with an AVF had lower PWV values and, therefore, lower arterial stiffness, which would, therefore, lower the serum endocan levels. In the existing literature, we did not find data on vascular access in relation to endocan levels and endothelial dysfunction.

The unexpectedly high prevalence of central venous catheters in this cohort likely reflects centre- and population-specific factors, including late referral to nephrology care: patients who begin dialysis without prior nephrology follow-up often start with a catheter due to the absence of a mature AVF or a graft. We also hypothesise that older patient populations with limited life expectancy or poor vascular access options may be maintained on catheters instead of undergoing AVF creation. In our study, it is evident that patients in the second and third tertiles (where CVCs are most prevalent), were statistically significantly older.

Among the parameters of peripheral and central haemodynamics, an important factor in progression of CVD and CKD is arterial stiffness. PWV has become a reliable indicator for evaluating arterial stiffness and serves as an independent predictor of cardiovascular and all-cause mortality in various populations, including those with ESKD [30–32]. We demonstrated that PWV increases with terciles of ndocan concentration, which aligns with the inter-related pathophysiological connection where endothelial dysfunction contributes to the development of arterial stiffness and vice versa. Similar findings have been reported in populations of patients with CKD, as well as in those on PD and HD [17,22,23]. Since endocan has been reported to affect CIMT and FMV [22,33], it is not surprising to observe a similar relationship with arterial stiffness.

In patients on HD without diabetes mellitus, the pathophysiological mechanisms driving CVEs may be less influenced by metabolic factors and more dependent on endothelial dysfunction, inflammation, and arterial stiffness, namely the pathways in which endocan is believed to play a role. Endocan reflects endothelial cell activation, a central feature in atherosclerosis, arterial stiffness, and vascular calcification, all of which are common in CKD and HD populations [23]. However, in non-diabetic patients, where glycaemic endothelial damage is absent, elevated endocan may more directly reflect non-metabolic endothelial injury (e.g., from uraemia, oxidative stress, fluid overload, or other mechanisms). Endocan modulates leukocyte adhesion and transmigration, promoting vascular inflammation, which is a known trigger for plaque instability and CVEs. This effect is independent of diabetic status and may be more pronounced in HD patients with a high inflammatory burden [22]. Studies suggest a link between elevated endocan levels and increased PWV, a surrogate marker of arterial stiffness and a strong independent predictor of cardiovascular mortality in HD patients [25]. In non-diabetic HD patients, elevated PWV and endocan may synergistically identify high-risk vascular phenotypes, even in the absence of traditional risk factors like hyperglycaemia.

The clinical application of endocan extends across several domains. As a marker of endothelial activation and vascular inflammation, endocan may serve in the early detection of subclinical vascular damage in high-risk groups such as patients with CKD, ESKD, diabetes, and hypertension. In the context of maintenance HD, where traditional risk markers often lack sensitivity, endocan may aid in risk stratification and longitudinal monitoring, providing insight into ongoing vascular injury. Additionally, given its correlation with arterial stiffness, endocan could be used as a complementary tool alongside PWV in the assessment of vascular aging. Also, its sensitivity to pro-inflammatory stimuli supports its potential role in monitoring systemic inflammation in CKD, ESKD, or autoimmune disease populations, where low-grade chronic inflammation significantly contributes to disease progression and adverse cardiovascular outcomes. Finally, it is important to mention the review article by Samouilidou et al. and the meta-analysis by Khalaji et al. which suggest that recent studies reveal that endocan could be a predictor of all-cause mortality and MACEs in CKD patients. Endocan levels were found to be higher in patients with CKD compared to healthy controls, despite high heterogeneity, and were also demonstrated as a negative prognostic factor in patients on HD, PD, and even after kidney transplantation [20,21].

Our study has several limitations, comparable to other studies in this field. Since the study was conducted at a single clinical centre and the exclusion criteria were strict, this resulted in a relatively small number of participants. Furthermore, it consisted only of Caucasian individuals, making extrapolation to other countries or populations partially limited. Additionally, we measured serum endocan levels only once, whereas serial monitoring of serum endocan levels may provide more prognostic information. In future studies, potential exclusion of medications that may interfere with endothelial integrity could also prove insightful. Despite these limitations, the unique focus on a non-diabetic population strengthens the relevance of these findings. We believe our study meaningfully contributes to the ever-expanding body of evidence linking serum endocan levels to CKD progression and adverse cardiovascular outcomes.

5. Conclusions

Our study explored and confirmed the association between elevated serum endocan levels in non-diabetic HD patients and the occurrence of MACEs and mortality and positions endocan as a cardiovascular risk factor, which can also serve as important biomarker reflecting endothelial dysfunction as a critical contributor to cardiovascular morbidity in ESKD. Conducting larger-scale, multicentre clinical trials that emphasise frequent follow-up could enhance our understanding of the applicability of endocan as a prognostic and diagnostic marker in kidney diseases, potentially even defining relevant cutoff values for its serum levels for timely identification of patients with the highest cardiovascular risk.

Author Contributions: Conceptualisation, M.Š. and D.M.; methodology, M.Š., D.M., and I.T.; project administration, M.Š. and D.M.; resources, M.Š., IŠ., and D.M.; software, E.O.; validation, I.Š., E.O., I.F., and M.P.; formal analysis, I.Š., E.O., I.F., and D.Š.; investigation, M.Š., M.P., I.T., and D.Š.; data curation, M.Š., M.P., and D.Š.; writing—original draft preparation, M.Š. and D.M.; writing—review and editing, D.M. and E.O.; visualisation, I.F. and I.T.; supervision, D.M. All authors have read and agreed to the published version of the manuscript.

Funding: This research received no external funding. The authors personally contributed financially to perform this study.

Institutional Review Board Statement: The study protocol adhered to the standards established by the latest revision of the Declaration of Helsinki and was approved by the Ethics Committee of the Faculty of Medicine Osijek and the Ethics Committee of the University Hospital Osijek (Number: R2-6782/2018, date of approval: 3 May 2018).

Informed Consent Statement: Informed consent was obtained from all subjects involved in the study.

Data Availability Statement: The dataset used, analysed, or generated in this research is available from the corresponding author (E.O.) upon reasonable request.

Acknowledgments: The authors are grateful to all the supporting staff and participants in our study for their time and cooperation.

Conflicts of Interest: The authors declare no conflicts of interest that may be perceived as inappropriately influencing the representation or interpretation of reported research results.

Abbreviations

The following abbreviations are used in this manuscript:

CKD	chronic kidney disease
CVD	cardiovascular disease
HD	haemodialysis
DKD	diabetes mellitus
MACE	major adverse cardiovascular event
AVF	arteriovenous fistulas
TCVC	tunnelled central venous catheter
ESKD	end-stage kidney disease
FMD	flow-mediated dilation
IgA	immunoglobulin A
PD	peritoneal dialysis
sICAM-1	intercellular adhesion molecule-1
sVCAM-1	vascular adhesion molecule-1
hs-CRP	high-sensitivity CRP
CIMT	carotid intima–media thickness
PWV	pulse wave velocity
AI	augmentation index
MAP	mean arterial pressure
PP	pulse pressure
SBP	systolic blood pressure
DBP	diastolic blood pressure
HR	heart rate

PTH	parathyroid hormone
BCM	bioimpedance method
ELISA	enzyme-linked immunosorbent assay
RAAS	renin angiotensin aldosterone system

References

1. Jha, V.; Garcia-Garcia, G.; Iseki, K.; Li, Z.; Naicker, S.; Plattner, B.; Saran, R.; Wang, A.Y.-M.; Yang, C.-W. Chronic kidney disease: Global dimension and perspectives. *Lancet* **2013**, *382*, 260–272. [CrossRef] [PubMed]
2. Wheeler, D.C. Cardiovascular disease in patients with chronic renal failure. *Lancet* **1996**, *348*, 1673–1674. [CrossRef] [PubMed]
3. Collins, A.J. Cardiovascular Mortality in End-Stage Renal Disease. *Am. J. Med. Sci.* **2003**, *325*, 163–167. [CrossRef] [PubMed]
4. National Institutes of Health; US Department of Health and Human Services. *United States Renal Data System. 2020 USRDS Annual Data Report: Epidemiology of Kidney Disease in the United States*; National Institutes of Health: Bethesda, MD, USA, 2020.
5. Makar, M.S.; Pun, P.H. Sudden Cardiac Death Among Hemodialysis Patients. *Am. J. Kidney Dis.* **2017**, *69*, 684–695. [CrossRef]
6. De Bie, M.K.; Van Dam, B.; Gaasbeek, A.; Van Buren, M.; Van Erven, L.; Bax, J.J.; Schalij, M.J.; Rabelink, T.J.; Jukema, J.W. The current status of interventions aiming at reducing sudden cardiac death in dialysis patients. *Eur. Heart J.* **2009**, *30*, 1559–1564. [CrossRef]
7. Herzog, C.A. Cardiac arrest in dialysis patients: Approaches to alter an abysmal outcome. *Kidney Int.* **2003**, *63*, S197–S200. [CrossRef]
8. Tri Tai Truyen, T.T.; Uy-Evanado, A.; Holmstrom, L.; Reinier, K.; Chugh, H.; Jui, J.; Herzog, C.A.; Chugh, S.S. Sudden Cardiac Arrest Associated with Hemodialysis: A Community-Based Study. Kidney360 [Internet]. 2025 January 17. Available online: https://journals.lww.com/10.34067/KID.0000000705 (accessed on 11 May 2025).
9. Umanath, K.; Lewis, J.B. Update on Diabetic Nephropathy: Core Curriculum 2018. *Am. J. Kidney Dis.* **2018**, *71*, 884–895. [CrossRef]
10. Sarnak, M.J.; Levey, A.S.; Schoolwerth, A.C.; Coresh, J.; Culleton, B.; Hamm, L.L.; McCullough, P.A.; Kasiske, B.L.; Kelepouris, E.; Klag, M.J.; et al. Kidney Disease as a Risk Factor for Development of Cardiovascular Disease: A Statement From the American Heart Association Councils on Kidney in Cardiovascular Disease, High Blood Pressure Research, Clinical Cardiology, and Epidemiology and Prevention. *Circulation* **2003**, *108*, 2154–2169. [CrossRef]
11. Liao, J.K. Linking endothelial dysfunction with endothelial cell activation. *J. Clin. Investig.* **2013**, *123*, 540–541. [CrossRef]
12. Alexander, Y.; Osto, E.; Schmidt-Trucksäss, A.; Shechter, M.; Trifunovic, D.; Duncker, D.J.; Aboyans, V.; Bäck, M.; Badimon, L.; Cosentino, F.; et al. Endothelial function in cardiovascular medicine: A consensus paper of the European Society of Cardiology Working Groups on Atherosclerosis and Vascular Biology, Aorta and Peripheral Vascular Diseases, Coronary Pathophysiology and Microcirculation, and Thrombosis. *Cardiovasc. Res.* **2021**, *117*, 29–42.
13. Bessa, J.; Albino-Teixeira, A.; Reina-Couto, M.; Sousa, T. Endocan: A novel biomarker for risk stratification, prognosis and therapeutic monitoring in human cardiovascular and renal diseases. *Clin. Chim. Acta* **2020**, *509*, 310–335. [CrossRef] [PubMed]
14. Sarrazin, S.; Adam, E.; Lyon, M.; Depontieu, F.; Motte, V.; Landolfi, C.; Lortat-Jacob, H.; Bechard, D.; Lassalle, P.; Delehedde, M. Endocan or endothelial cell specific molecule-1 (ESM-1): A potential novel endothelial cell marker and a new target for cancer therapy. *Biochim. Biophys. Acta BBA—Rev. Cancer* **2006**, *1765*, 25–37. [CrossRef] [PubMed]
15. Afsar, B.; Takir, M.; Kostek, O.; Covic, A.; Kanbay, M. Endocan: A New Molecule Playing a Role in the Development of Hypertension and Chronic Kidney Disease? *J. Clin. Hypertens.* **2014**, *16*, 914–916. [CrossRef]
16. Samouilidou, E.; Bountou, E.; Papandroulaki, F.; Papamanolis, M.; Papakostas, D.; Grapsa, E. Serum Endocan Levels are Associated With Paraoxonase 1 Concentration in Patients With Chronic Kidney Disease. *Ther. Apher. Dial.* **2018**, *22*, 325–331. [CrossRef]
17. Poon, P.Y.K.; Ng, J.K.C.; Fung, W.W.S.; Chow, K.M.; Kwan, B.C.H.; Li, P.K.T.; Szeto, C.-C. Relationship between Plasma Endocan Level and Clinical Outcome of Chinese Peritoneal Dialysis Patients. *Kidney Blood Press. Res.* **2019**, *44*, 1259–1270. [CrossRef]
18. Balta, S.; Mikhailidis, D.P.; Demirkol, S.; Ozturk, C.; Celik, T.; Iyisoy, A. Endocan: A novel inflammatory indicator in cardiovascular disease? *Atherosclerosis* **2015**, *243*, 339–343. [CrossRef]
19. Malyszko, J.; Koc-Żórawska, E.; Malyszko, J.S. Endocan Concentration in Kidney Transplant Recipients. *Transplant. Proc.* **2018**, *50*, 1798–1801. [CrossRef]
20. Khalaji, A.; Behnoush, A.H.; Mohtasham Kia, Y.; Alehossein, P.; Bahiraie, P. High circulating endocan in chronic kidney disease? A systematic review and meta-analysis. Battaglia Y, editor. *PLoS ONE* **2023**, *18*, e0289710. [CrossRef]
21. Samouilidou, E.; Athanasiadou, V.; Grapsa, E. Prognostic and Diagnostic Value of Endocan in Kidney Diseases. *Int. J. Nephrol.* **2022**, *2022*, 3861092. [CrossRef]
22. Yilmaz, M.I.; Siriopol, D.; Saglam, M.; Kurt, Y.G.; Unal, H.U.; Eyileten, T.; Gok, M.; Cetinkaya, H.; Oguz, Y.; Sari, S.; et al. Plasma endocan levels associate with inflammation, vascular abnormalities, cardiovascular events, and survival in chronic kidney disease. *Kidney Int.* **2014**, *86*, 1213–1220. [CrossRef]

23. Kim, J.S.; Ko, G.J.; Kim, Y.G.; Lee, S.Y.; Lee, D.Y.; Jeong, K.H.; Lee, S.H. Plasma Endocan as a Predictor of Cardiovascular Event in Patients with End-Stage Renal Disease on Hemodialysis. *J. Clin. Med.* **2020**, *9*, 4086. [CrossRef] [PubMed]
24. Lin, J.H.; Hsu, B.G.; Wang, C.H.; Tsai, J.P. Endocan as a Potential Marker for Predicting All-Cause Mortality in Hemodialysis Patients. *J. Clin. Med.* **2023**, *12*, 7427. [CrossRef] [PubMed]
25. Wu, T.J.; Wang, C.H.; Lai, Y.H.; Kuo, C.H.; Lin, Y.L.; Hsu, B.G. Serum Endocan Is a Risk Factor for Aortic Stiffness in Patients Undergoing Maintenance Hemodialysis. *Medicina* **2024**, *60*, 984. [CrossRef]
26. Malyszko, J. Mechanism of endothelial dysfunction in chronic kidney disease. *Clin. Chim. Acta* **2010**, *411*, 1412–1420. [CrossRef]
27. Qiu, C.R.; Fu, Q.; Sui, J.; Zhang, Q.; Wei, P.; Wu, Y.; Zhu, K.; Lu, Y.; Zong, B. Serum Endothelial Cell–Specific Molecule 1 (Endocan) Levels in Patients With Acute Myocardial Infarction and Its Clinical Significance: A Pilot Study. *Angiology* **2017**, *68*, 354–359. [CrossRef]
28. Whayne, T.F. Endocan in Hypertension and Cardiovascular Disease. *Angiology* **2014**, *65*, 757–759. [CrossRef]
29. Pawlak, K.; Mysliwiec, M.; Pawlak, D. Endocan—the new endothelial activation marker independently associated with soluble endothelial adhesion molecules in uraemic patients with cardiovascular disease. *Clin. Biochem.* **2015**, *48*, 425–430. [CrossRef]
30. Blacher, J.; Safar, M.E.; Guerin, A.P.; Pannier, B.; Marchais, S.J.; London, G.M. Aortic pulse wave velocity index and mortality in end-stage renal disease. *Kidney Int.* **2003**, *63*, 1852–1860. [CrossRef]
31. Laurent, S.; Cockcroft, J.; Van Bortel, L.; Boutouyrie, P.; Giannattasio, C.; Hayoz, D.; Pannier, B.; Vlachopoulos, C.; Wilkinson, I.; Struijker-Boudier, H. Expert consensus document on arterial stiffness: Methodological issues and clinical applications. *Eur. Heart J.* **2006**, *27*, 2588–2605. [CrossRef]
32. Vlachopoulos, C.; Aznaouridis, K.; Stefanadis, C. Prediction of Cardiovascular Events and All-Cause Mortality With Arterial Stiffness. *J. Am. Coll. Cardiol.* **2010**, *55*, 1318–1327. [CrossRef]
33. Lu, Q.; Cheng, L.T.; Wang, T.; Wan, J.; Liao, L.L.; Zeng, J.; Qin, C.; Li, K.-J. Visceral Fat, Arterial Stiffness, and Endothelial Function in Peritoneal Dialysis Patients. *J. Ren. Nutr.* **2008**, *18*, 495–502. [CrossRef]

MDPI AG
Grosspeteranlage 5
4052 Basel
Switzerland
Tel.: +41 61 683 77 34

Medicina Editorial Office
E-mail: medicina@mdpi.com
www.mdpi.com/journal/medicina

www.ingramcontent.com/pod-product-compliance
Lightning Source LLC
Chambersburg PA
CBHW062102220926
51850CB00010B/2863
* 9 7 8 3 7 2 5 8 5 7 1 7 3 *